WORKING IN ORBIT AND BEYOND:
THE CHALLENGES FOR SPACE MEDICINE

AAS PRESIDENT
 E. Larry Heacock   NOAA/NESS

VICE PRESIDENT - PUBLICATIONS
 Walter Froehlich   International Science Writers

SERIES EDITOR
 Dr. Horace Jacobs   Univelt, Incorporated

EDITORS
 David B. Lorr   Space Medicine Systems, Incorporated
 Dr. Victoria Garshnek   The George Washington University
 Dr. Claude Cadoux   Union Memorial Hospital, Balitmore, MD

ASSOCIATE EDITOR
 Robert H. Jacobs   Univelt, Incorporated

Thanks are due Carmen Martinez-Ivins and Doreen L. Linnan, Univelt, Inc., for final preparation of the manuscript for publication.

Front Cover Illustration:

Ross, anchored to foot restraint on RMS, works with ACCESS. Photo was taken by Spring with 35 mm camera. Crewmembers for the week-long flight were astronauts Brewster Shaw, Jr., Bryan D. O'Connor, Mary L. Cleave, Sherwood C. Spring, Jerry L. Ross and payload specialists Rodolfo Neri of Mexico and Charles D. Walker of McDonnell Douglas. The mission launched from KSC on November 26, 1985 and landed at Edwards Air Force Base on December 3 (NASA Photo Nos. 85-H-534, 85-HC-483, and 61B-102-022).

Frontispiece:

Space Art - "Spacelab 1", oil painting by Charles Schmidt. NASA and ESA astronauts and technicians work on the scientific laboratory during Mission Sequence Tests, in preparation for the first Spacelab Mission, STS-9, launched from NASA/KSC, November 28, 1983. This painting was especially commissioned to present to the European Space Agency for exhibition in Paris. NASA Art Program, September 16, 1983 - Art size: 52 inches by 72 inches (NASA Photo Nos. 83-H-799 and 83-HC-677).

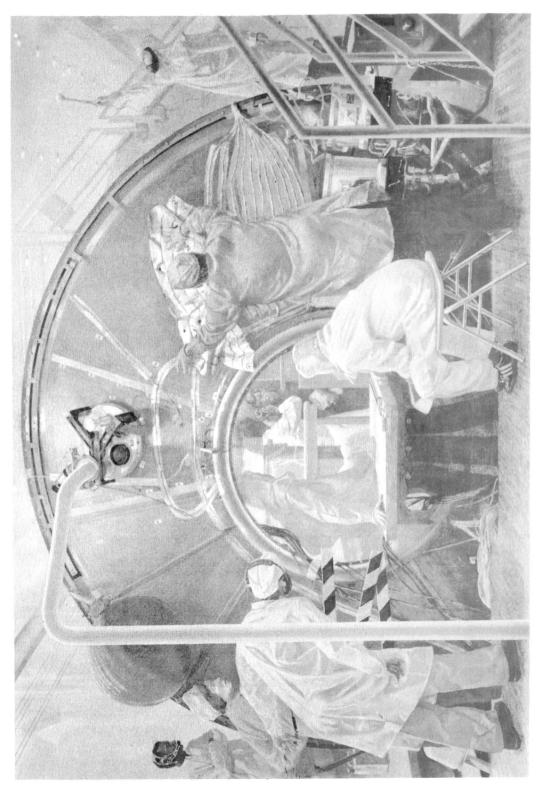

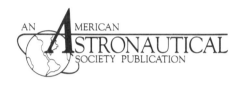

WORKING IN ORBIT AND BEYOND: THE CHALLENGES FOR SPACE MEDICINE

Edited by
David B. Lorr
Victoria Garshnek
Claude Cadoux

Volume 72
SCIENCE AND TECHNOLOGY SERIES
A Supplement to Advances in the Astronautical Sciences

This proceedings volume is based on a course sponsored by the Georgetown University Department of Continuing Medical Education held June 20-21, 1987, Washington, D.C.

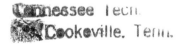
*Published for the American Astronautical Society by
Univelt, Incorporated, P.O. Box 28130, San Diego, California 92128*

Affiliated with the American Association for the Advancement of Science
Member of the International Astronautical Federation

First Printing 1989

ISSN 0278-4017

ISBN 0-87703-295-5 (Hard Cover)
ISBN 0-87703-296-3 (Soft Cover)

Published for the American Astronautical Society
by Univelt, Inc., P.O. Box 28130, San Diego, California 92128

Printed and Bound in the U.S.A.

FOREWORD

This proceedings volume is based on the course entitled, "Working in Orbit and Beyond: The Challenges for Space Medicine". It was sponsored by the Georgetown University Department of Continuing Medical Education and held on June 20-21, 1987.

The objective of the program was to increase the medical community's awareness of the problems and solutions particular to space medicine and to facilitate the dissemination of this information to other interested personnel.

The course description included: the differences in normal physiology and adaptation to zero gravity, the special hazards of life and work in space, their countermeasures, and future challenges in space medicine.

Special thanks for support of the program must be given to Dr. Ronald White and Barbara Lujan of the NASA Life Sciences Division, Dr. Thomas Stair from the Georgetown University Department of Continuing Medical Education, and the program speakers who generously gave of their time and efforts.

Finally, the Lockheed Engineering and Management Services Company, Inc. and the Sophron Foundation should be recognized for their financial contributions.

David B. Lorr
Victoria Garshnek
Claude Cadoux

CONTENTS

AAS 87-152

CURRENT STATUS AND FUTURE DIRECTION OF NASA'S SPACE LIFE SCIENCES PROGRAM

Ronald J. White and Barbara F. Lujan[*]

This paper summarizes the current status and future directions of a portion of NASA's Life Sciences Program. Only those elements of the program related to manned space flight and biological scientific studies in space are covered in this brief summary.

INTRODUCTION

There is little doubt that the ubiquitous force of gravity has dictated the internal and external shape of life on Earth in ways which are, at the same time, both dramatic and subtle. Gravity not only preceded life on Earth, but also has been a pervasive and stable companion of evolution for all of the eons of existence of life, whatever its form. An organism's ability to perceive gravity, to interpret correctly the relationship between gravity and its position, and to make physical adjustments necessary to prevent damage in a threatening situation frequently determines if the organism will survive to maturity. All life appears to be molded and constrained by gravity, and the relationship between gravity and life is so intimate that, prior to the advent of space flight, no one could predict precisely how, or even whether, any particular biological process would function in the virtual absence of gravity. With the passage of time and the accumulation of data, a new field of scientific research, space life sciences, has been born.

Given the uncertainty that existed in the days before manned orbital flights concerning how biological processes would function without gravity, it should come as no surprise that biological experimentation in space preceded man's visit to that environment. Bacteria, fungi, various cell cultures, plants, dogs, and monkeys all flew in space before man. In 1961, the first man in space carried a package containing bacteria with him, pocket mice journeyed with man to the Moon and back in 1972, and man has continued to carry ever more complicated scientific investigations of biological significance on the spacecraft he uses. In addition, both the United States and the Soviet Union have flown dedicated biological satellites, but only the Soviet Union has maintained a regular flight program of such spacecraft, with flights every two or three years. Many of the early biological experiments in space were crude by scientific standards and were designed to address questions of survivability and gross function in the space environment. As data from these early flights accumulated and were analyzed, it became clear that there were no biological surprises. Space flight,

* Life Sciences Division, NASA Headquarters, 600 Independence Avenue, S.W., Washington, D.C. 20546.

1

in general, turned out to be essentially benign and tolerable. Cellular effects were subtle, and thus difficult to detect, but at the level of more complex organisms, with developed systems for sensing and maintaining their orientation with respect to gravity, there were significant effects. Thus, for both plant and animal systems, the key scientific questions became: how does the organism perceive gravity, how is that information transmitted to a site capable of responding to the perception, and how does the responding site process the information and control the response itself? In addition, it became increasingly clear that a key question concerned the role of gravity in the life cycle of an organism. Does gravity's influence extend even into the initial days or hours of life, how does gravity affect the development of a seed or embryo, or the maturation and behavior of the organism? Such questions formed the basis for many of the studies of the 1980s. Finally, as space research tools became better developed, and as more sensitive research techniques were introduced into the laboratory, the question of determining the subtle cellular responses to space flight was re-introduced.

Man, like every other organism on Earth, is completely adapted to the normal gravitational force which exists at the surface of our planet. There are only a very few moments during most of our lives on Earth when this force does not act on the body (e.g., during some sports activities such as jumping on a trampoline, or when flying in an airplane during a parabolic trajectory), but the duration of such exceptions is extremely short. During a space flight, the effective force of gravity decreases to a thousandth or a millionth of its normal value, and investigating life and the adaptation of biological systems in such an altered environment is both highly interesting and extremely important, particularly if man is ever to journey for long periods in space.

Data gathered over the years suggest the following broad picture of the human physiological responses to the microgravity environment of space flight. Disturbances in the cardiovascular, fluid-electrolyte, erythropoietic, musculoskeletal, and metabolic systems, which are found during and after space flight, appear to be attributed to at least two major effects of weightlessness. First, the absence of hydrostatic forces results in redistribution of the body fluids in a manner favoring upper body hypervolemia. Correction of this disturbance by the fluid regulating systems leads to a reduction in extra-cellular fluids, most important of which is the blood volume. Second, the absence of deformation forces results in degradation of normally load-bearing tissues with the major consequence being a reduction of intracellular constituents of bone and muscle mass. In addition, there appears to be a long-term alteration of the metabolic state. This alteration is partly reflected by changes in dietary intake and is influenced by exercise levels and by weightlessness itself, in some undefined manner. For example, a diminished dietary intake (both voluntary and involuntary) appears to be implicated, at least partially, in the loss of fat stores, muscle tissue, body water, and red cell mass, as well as in altered hormonal secretion and renal excretion. The stress of space flight also plays a role in man's response and this is reflected by significant increases in cortisol levels, which have widespread metabolic consequences. The occurrence of space motion sickness early in the flight and other vestibular disturbances manifested upon one-g recovery may be related to the headward displacement of body fluids, possible temporary morphological changes in the vestibular apparatus, and, perhaps most importantly, conflicting cues from multiple sensory stimuli. Whatever the cause of space motion sickness, it is associated with a significant voluntary reduction in food and fluid consumption with the possibility of wide-ranging physiological consequences, at least during the early period of flight. All of these events have both acute and long-term effects which lead to the notable and consistent findings of loss in weight, change in body composition, altered blood biochemistry, and, upon return to a one-g environment, decreased tolerance for orthostasis and a temporarily compromised response to physical activity.

With few exceptions, findings to date suggest that the responses of the body to space flight are not pathological in nature. Rather, these responses can be considered appropriate and effective adaptations to the nearly weightless environment. Many of the effects which have been observed can be tentatively explained in terms of normal, although complex, feedback regulatory processes. Upon return to a one-g environment, some dysfunction may appear because the functioning level of adaptation reached in zero-g is inappropriate to normal gravitational loading. However, following a short period of readaptation these changes appear reversible, at least for the time span over which man has been studied in space.

CURRENT PROGRAM

The current NASA Life Sciences Flight Experiments Program contains over 60 scientific investigations covering a broad spectrum of fundamental and applied research areas. Mission assignments on presently scheduled Spacelab missions (including Spacelab Life Sciences 1 and 2, International Microgravity Laboratory 1, and Spacelab J) have been made for over 30 of these investigations. It is impossible to summarize all of these studies in this paper. The currently assigned investigations involve interdisciplinary, multi-species (using humans, laboratory rats, and squirrel monkeys) studies of the early and short-term adaptive responses to space flight and readaptation to Earth, animal model validation studies, and a number of basic gravitational biology studies (using plants, small animals, and cellular systems). For example, in the cardiovascular and related renal-endocrine areas, parallel studies in humans, rats, and monkeys will examine, in detail, the overall cardiopulmonary and fluid/electrolyte adjustments to zero-g by examining closely connected individual elements of the circulatory system, the capillary beds, the autonomic mechanisms, the heart, the lung, the body fluid volumes, and the major fluid and salt regulating hormones. Plant experiments will study geotropic and phototropic responses to weightlessness. Frog studies will examine the effect of gravity on the symmetry of developing amphibian embryos by flying male and female frogs in space and observing the early development of frog eggs following inflight fertilization.

FUTURE DIRECTIONS

Life Sciences research in space has progressed to the point where we understand, in a general way, the challenges which space flight presents to living systems.

In a limited number of disciplines, we are able to focus on potential mechanisms associated with the gross physiological and biological changes which have been observed during and following space flight. But, the prospect of an extended human presence in space in the Space Station era, and, in the early 21st century, manned bases on the Moon and Mars, raises serious questions about human adaptability to the space environment. Crewmembers have returned in good health after three months in space, and have performed extravehicular activity (EVA) as hazardous and taxing as satellite capture and repair. Nevertheless, the achievement of a permanent presence in space presents a new array of biomedical, psychological, and human engineering challenges and opportunities, as well as problems and hazards. In this paper, we will summarize a number of the life sciences issues related to supporting an extended human presence in space. Programs to address these issues are being developed at the present time.

Many of the biomedical issues considered in the light of long-duration space flight relate to the effects of ambient characteristics of space on living systems. Specifically, attention must be given to the deconditioning of physiological systems which have evolved in gravity, increased exposure to solar and cosmic radiation beyond the protection of Earth's atmosphere and geomagnetic field, the remoteness from such ground resources as adequate medical care, a regenerative life support environment, and the ramifications in a limited living space for toxic buildup and psychological stress. Moreover, the capability for optimum performance implies more than simple survival; it includes the development of productive tools for maximizing crew performance and a living environment which minimizes the psychological stresses of isolation and confinement. Medical data from Skylab and Space Shuttle have demonstrated the types of physiological alterations that may be expected in the course of space flight. Space medicine has progressed to the point where medical care can be designed and delivered with reasonable confidence on Shuttle flights, including polar missions, and for 90-day tours of duty on Space Station. However, the missions envisioned for the next decade and the early 21st century will involve significantly longer stays in space. As missions move away from Earth, the current reliance on medical support on the ground will become untenable. Further development of inflight diagnostic capabilities, preventive medicine, and countermeasures is essential to ensure the safety of humans undertaking a manned mission to Mars or manning a permanent lunar base.

Missions exceeding several months must ensure not only crew survival, but crew productivity and safe readaptation to the gravity field of Earth. U.S. and Soviet programs have shown that the most important physiological issues are bone demineralization, muscle atrophy, changes in the cardiovascular, pulmonary, immune, endocrine, and vestibular systems, and alterations in bone marrow, renal, and neurologic function. Not all of these issues can be resolved by ground-based research or by short Shuttle flights. Early experimentation on Space Station laboratories is essential to properly understand the process by which humans adapt to long-term stays in microgravity and readapt to Earth's one-g environment. Variable-gravity facilities will also be required for studying the partial-gravity effects of the Moon and Mars, as well as for determining the necessity and efficacy of artificial gravity as a countermeasure.

The central issue of space radiation is the danger to the safety and health of humans posed by radiation during long-term missions in space. Although it has been estimated that a Mars mission can be accomplished with nominal radiation exposure to a crew (about half of the current lifetime limit of industrial workers), the stochastic effects of certain high-energy ions are not well understood. In addition, major solar flare events could pose a lethal threat to interplanetary travelers. Hence, to properly prepare for such missions, it will be necessary to expand the current radiation research program in the areas of shielding strategies, biologic effects, and therapeutical countermeasures. All missions outside of the Earth's protective magnetosphere will also require a solar radiation warning system and safe haven for the crew.

A breathable atmosphere and potable water supply are critical to the well-being of humans who live and work in space for long periods of time, whether in spacecraft or on the surface of the Moon or Mars. Continual habitation, materials processing, and biological and other experimental activities increase the probability of the release of potentially harmful chemical and biologic contaminants into closed environments. Volatile, dissolved, particulate, and microbial contaminants must be consistently monitored in the spacecraft and habitats used during long-term missions. Assuring the quality of the recycled atmosphere and water during these missions will require development of new environmental standards, purification technologies, and alarm systems.

Spacecraft and planetary habitat life support systems will have different requirements with regard to technology and the degree of recycling nutrients. The necessity of a life support system with living components for a spacecraft is dependent on design criteria such as weight and space. However, a closed ecological life support system is vital for extended manned activity on lunar or Martian bases. Planetary environments may provide such essentials as water, oxygen, carbon dioxide, and an inert substrate for the life support cycle, whereas spacecraft systems must be totally autonomous. Although much development is necessary to achieve an operational closed life support system, a hybrid system using crop plants and physical and chemical technologies could be designed by the end of the century. Secondary microbial food processing, algal protein production, and waste recycling will probably require technological development and a substantially longer period of research and development.

Optimal crew performance is critical for both crew survival and for maintaining the high productivity required during interplanetary missions. Due to the complexity of tasks and communication delays with Earth, space operations will have significant autonomy and many artificial intelligence elements. Considerable attention must therefore be given to human operator interaction with onboard computers, robots, and telepresence systems. In virtually all instances in which humans interact with complex, technology-intensive systems, human error has become a serious consideration in system design. Such errors can be significantly reduced by research and work station design and verification, and by computer simulations of human interactive systems.

Social and psychological tensions causing counterproductive behavior have been observed within small crews maintained in confined environments for extended periods. However, these problems are minor in comparison with those that may be elicited by the stresses of a long Mars mission. Behavior and mental problems could have a catastrophic impact on mission success. Behavioral research is required to optimize crew selection, compatibility, performance, training, recreation, privacy, and chain of command. Such research should include experiments in authentic analog environments, such as undersea habitats, as well as longitudinal studies of Shuttle and Space Station crews.

In a microgravity environment, where there is almost no gravity, where convection almost disappears, where stratification of layers decreases significantly, and where surface tension dominates, one may anticipate major impacts on metabolic processes which may be manifest in subtle ways. Such impacts may be reflected in the genesis of the shape and form of cells, tissues and organs. Since shape and form is tightly linked to physiology, perturbations in shape and form will have significance for the distribution and partitioning of fluids and solutes within cells and tissues, and, ultimately, the whole body of plants and animals. Gravity is an asymmetric stimulus on Earth. Asymmetry is a dominant feature of plants and animals, from the cellular level up to the entire organism level. A fundamental question in basic gravitational biology to be answered in the future is how dependent is the asymmetry of living things on the asymmetric stimulus of gravity. Other questions can be asked. What is the role of gravity in the evolution of bilateral symmetry, anterior and posterior ends, and dorso-ventral organization of body parts? What is the role of gravity in shaping the gravity-sensing systems (bioaccelerometers) in a comparative series of animals? At the heart of such questions is the issue of the level of interaction between genetic direction and environmental influence, a major and significant question in biology today. Similar questions arise when dealing with plants. As cells develop in a multi-cellular plant, they become morphologically and functionally different from one another, even though they contain identical genetic information. The mechanism of this cell differentiation is one of the most provocative problems of modern biology. The question is whether gravity plays a determinative role in this differentiation by affecting the relative position of the cells to one another or by affecting the constituents within the cells. Must plants have a gravity vector, and if so, of what size and direction, in order for normal development to occur generation after generation?

CONCLUSION

In this paper, the current status and future directions of NASA's Life Sciences Program are briefly summarized. The life sciences are intricately woven into the fabric of the technological world enfolding the space program, and they contribute strongly to the overall list of benefits to be derived from man's journey into space. Elements of the life sciences are involved in determining the most productive use of man in the space environment, in the design of habitable manned facilities, in the determination of the types of systems required to support the various facets of man, in the maintenance of good health, and in the care of man during sickness and injury. Other components of the life sciences seek to use the unique environment of space as a tool to probe some of the mysteries of life, particularly regarding how living things perceive and react to gravity. The ultimate value of such research to man is difficult to estimate, but there is no way to learn more about the effects of gravity on living things or to extend the ability of man to stay in space without leaving the surface of the Earth. The questions which could be answered are important enough to warrant the effort.

VESTIBULAR FACTORS INFLUENCING THE BIOMEDICAL SUPPORT OF HUMANS IN SPACE

Byron K. Lichtenberg[*]

This paper describes the biomedical support aspects of humans in space with respect to the vestibular system. The vestibular system is thought to be the primary sensory system involved in the short-term effects of space motion sickness although there is increasing evidence that many factors play a role in this complex set of symptoms. There is the possibility that an individual's inner sense of orientation may be strongly coupled with the susceptibility to space motion sickness. A variety of suggested counter-measures for space motion sickness is described. Although there are no known ground-based tests that can predict space motion sickness, the search should go on.

The long-term effects of the vestibular system in weightlessness are still relatively unknown. Some preliminary data have shown that the otoconia are irregular in size and distribution following extended periods of weight-lessness.

The ramifications of these data are not yet known and because the data were obtained on lower order animals, definitive studies and results must wait until the Space Station era when higher primates can be studied for long-duration flights.

This leads us to artificial gravity, the last topic of this paper. The vestibular system is intimately tied to this question since it has been shown on Earth that exposure to a slow rotating room causes motion sickness for some period of time before adaptation occurs. If the artificial gravity is intermit-tent, will this mean that people will get sick every time they experience it? The data from many astronauts return to Earth indicate that a variety of sensory illusions are present, especially immediately upon return to the 1 g environment. Oscillopsia or apparent motion of the visual surroundings upon head motion along with inappropriate eye motions for a given head motion all indicate that there is much to be studied yet about the ves-tibular and CNS systems reaction to a sudden application of a steady state acceleration field like 1 g.

From the above information it is obvious that the vestibular system does have unique requirements when it comes to the biomedical support of space flight. This is not to say that other areas such as cardio-vascular, musculo-skeletal, immunological and hematological systems don't have their own unique requirements but that possible solutions to one system can provide continuing problems to another system. For example, artifi-cial gravity might be helpful for long-term stabilization of bone demineralization or cardio-vascular deconditioning but might introduce a

---

* Dr. Lichtenberg is President of Payload Systems, Inc., 66 Central Street, Wellesley, Massachusetts 02181.

new set of problems in orientation, vestibular conflict and just plain body motion in a rotating space vehicle.

KEYWORDS: Vestibular system; space biomedicine; space adaptation syndrome; artificial gravity on Space Station.

INTRODUCTION

The topic of biomedical support of humans is very broad and encompasses such areas as environmental control systems, radiation protection, cardio-vascular stimulation, musculo-skeletal maintenance, immunological system responses, human factors, behavior and psychology, and the vestibular system. This paper will address only the vestibular system and will divide the effects of weightlessness on the system into short-term (several weeks to several months) and long-term (over about six months) effects. These dividing lines are not firm but rather stem from our current knowledge that there are short-term vestibular adaptation effects that occur on the order of 3-4 days and then the system seems to reach a new operating condition. For the long-term designation, we have very little information but it appears that any potential change in the system over the long-term must take months to years to occur.

The vestibular system exists primarily to provide orientation ability, to stabilize our eyes during head and body motion, and to help control posture and locomotion. It consists of two sub-systems, the semicircular canals which sense primarily angular accelerations (yaw, pitch and roll) of the head; and the otolith organs which sense primarily linear accelerations, one of which is the Earth's gravity. It is impossible for the otoliths to distinguish between gravity and other linear accelerations. For example, to distinguish between a head tilt (left or right) with respect to Earth's vertical and an acceleration to the left or right, one must use the semicircular canals to sense the rotation of the head which gives the cue that a head tilt has taken place. When a person goes into orbit, which will henceforth be called microgravity, the net linear acceleration (gravity minus the centripetal acceleration of the spacecraft) is effectively zero.

SHORT-TERM EFFECTS

There are several short-term effects of microgravity on the vestibular system. These include charges in orientation ability, apparent motion of the visual field, and reinterpretation of the sensory input generated by motion in the space vehicle. These phenomena can produce space motion sickness in many of the people that travel in space.

Space Motion Sickness

In microgravity, when a person moves his head in yaw, pitch or roll, the semicircular canals sense this rotation but the otoliths detect only a low-level short-term linear acceleration because these sensors are not located exactly at the center of rotation of the head. These signals are different from the inputs generated on the Earth.

When a person translates (moves side to side, forward-backward, or headward-footward) the only signals are transient linear accelerations sensed by the otoliths.

The first clue that something is different from Earth (with respect to the sensory system) is that about 50% of the space travelers seem to be susceptible to space motion sickness. We believe that this sickness is correlated to head motions. It is hypothesized that sensory conflict occurs when a crewmember moves in the vehicle. In this case, the otoliths sense no change in static orientation (because the gravity vector is nulled), but the semicircular canals and eyes still give correct information about pitch, yaw and roll. This induces a variety of symptoms of which some are similar to ground-based motion sickness and some are different.

Over several days, the brain learns to reinterpret the output of the otoliths as being a true transient linear acceleration of the body (left-right, up-down, fore-aft) and not connected at all with a roll or static head tilt (the way it does on Earth). Only when the brain senses semicircular canal stimulation does it decide that a true head roll or angular motion has taken place. The phenomenon is called the otolith tilt-translation reinterpretation hypothesis (OTTR) and will be discussed more in the return-to-Earth phenomena section.

The biomedical support needed to help ease the first 3-4 days of microgravity extends from practical advice on how to minimize symptoms and what to do if symptoms appear, to what precautions should be taken by other crewmembers, to advice on treatment such as drug usage, hydration patterns, and activity levels. Because it is strongly indicated that head motions play a major part in the onset of space motion sickness, the first suggestion is to limit head motions during the first several days, or at least move slowly. Because there is a delay between the head motion activity and the onset of symptoms, one must realize that when symptoms occur, there will be a corresponding delay between the time that head motions are restricted and the time that symptoms decay. Usually, 15 to 20 minutes of no or limited head motion is sufficient to reduce the symptoms.

For many people, seeing another crewmember in an unusual orientation can be provocative. Therefore, it is important that if one or more people on board are suffering, the other crewmembers should make every effort to maintain the same orientation so that unusual or unexpected visual scenes are avoided. Similarly, outside views of the Earth can be provocative so that sightseeing might be delayed until several days into the flight.

Although one of the symptoms of space motion sickness usually is loss of appetite, it is suggested that crewmembers attempt to drink as much water as possible in order to avoid dehydration problems that can complicate the space adaptation syndrome. Finally, it is clear that people suffering from space motion sickness should not be scheduled for Extra-Vehicular Activity (EVA) during the first several days of the flight. In fact, first-time space travelers and people that have experienced space motion sickness on previous flights should delay EVAs until several days into the flight.

Most ground-based motion sickness susceptibility tests can't predict who will get sick in space or help adapt people prior to their entry onto orbit. In the past several years, however, experiments indicate that there might be a slight correlation between a person's susceptibility to left-right reversing prism goggles and space motion sickness susceptibility. Due to the small number of subjects tested so far, no statistically significant conclusions can be reached yet. The search for ground-based stimuli that can either predict or help adapt people before flight should continue however. The object should not be to preselect crewmembers but to better identify the mechanisms so that potential ground-based adaptation measures can be taken to help ease the discomfort of the first several days in orbit. These measures may be even more important when large numbers of non-professional astronauts travel in space in the not-too-distant future. This statement does not imply that professional astronauts are any less susceptible or any more able to cope with space motion sickness, only that it would be nice if the tourist bus that will someday operate routinely to and from space could spare its occupants some measure of discomfort.

There is anecdotal evidence that indicates there might be some correlation between people's mental image of themselves in space with respect to their surroundings (either the inside of a spacecraft or the Earth) and their space motion sickness susceptibility. On several flights now, when the question was asked about how a person orients to the inside of the vehicle, the answer falls into two categories. The first answer is, "I take my orientation cues from the visual world (orbiter, Spacelab, or Earth)" The second answer is, "I don't care where the visual scene is, my feet are 'down' and I am prepared to accept any orientation with respect to the vehicle or Earth."

The interpretation of the above information is not totally straightforward when it is compared with the results of tests of field dependence on crewmembers. A standard test of field dependence is the rod and frame test. This test (done on Earth) measures the ability of a subject to set a line to the vertical first with no outside visual cues (done in a dark room with a luminous line), and then with a lighted frame that can be tilted with respect to the vertical. A field-dependent person would tend to be influenced by his visual surroundings and thus move the line away from the vertical towards the frame orientation. There are data emerging that indicate that the sensation of orientation is not connected to field dependence however. For example, on *Spacelab 1,* the most field-dependent person was the one who most believed his own body orientation (feet were "down") and was able to accept any orientation of the vehicle. This person was premedicated and didn't experience any motion sickness symptoms. Another crewmember on the flight who was also premedicated but did not have the ability to "move" the vehicle to his own orientation did get sick. Two other crewmembers that did not premedicate did experience symptoms and both relied mainly on the vehicle orientation for their own orientation. On D-1, the person who was least susceptible to space motion sickness also experienced the least dependence on the interior visual orientation. Conversely, several who were the sickest took the visual orientation of the vehicle as the major influence in determining their own orientation.

In the short-term, the most important effect of the vestibular adaptation to microgravity is that the space motion sickness that usually persists 3 to 4 days, subsides and there appears to be a greatly enhanced immunity against such motion-producing stimuli like out-of-plane head motions during constant rotation, rapid pitching motions of the head, and visual field disturbances such as encountering the Earth in an unanticipated orientation, or working next to an upside-down crewmember. While in space this adaptation to a new set of sensory inputs is very beneficial but can cause problems upon return to Earth's gravity.

Return-to-Earth Phenomena

Upon reentry into the Earth's atmosphere after adaptation to microgravity, the effects of a net acceleration to the otoliths are noticed at a very early stage. Even when the total acceleration is on the order of 0.75 g, there are several sensations that need to be understood and accounted for. First, when a crewmember rolls his head left-right, an inappropriate visual compensation occurs which is perceived not only as a roll of the visual field, but also a slewing of the visual field horizontally. This has been called the otolith tilt-translation reinterpretation hypothesis and is interpreted as follows: In space after several days, the brain learns that head angular motions are signaled only by the semicircular canals; the otoliths don't change their output. When the otoliths are stimulated, this is due to a translation. After return to Earth, with even small head motions away from the vertical (small enough so that the semicircular canals are not stimulated), the otoliths receive linear acceleration stimuli from gravity. The brain interprets this as a translation and drives eye motions to compensate for the perceived translation. Because the small head rolls, with respect to gravity, can be either left-right or up-down, the sensation is one of the entire world moving in two dimensions. This leads to postural instability and difficulty in walking in the dark.

This sensation needs to be understood for the safety of flight aspects of operating the orbiter during the reentry and landing phase. If a malfunction dictates a rapid head motion to search for a switch or circuit breaker on either an overhead panel or one aft of the pilot's seats, then oscillopsia (perceived motion of the visual field) can occur. This means that there is blurring and reduced visual acuity, both of which can be a problem if not anticipated. Second, thresholds of motion detection can be altered and thus change the pilot's sensation and control inputs. Changes in pitch rate sensation of the orbiter during landing, and deceleration during braking are just two of the areas that need to be investigated.

Postural instability immediately after landing and upon egress needs to be better studied so that crewmembers can understand these effects and take them into account. This is especially critical if an emergency evacuation is required and/or the orbiter loses electrical power and the cabin is dark during egress. Experiments to date have shown that there are changes in the reflex loops such as a reduction in ocular counter-rolling (driven by the vestibular system), postural instability as measured by the sharpened Romberg test, the rails test, and several tilt platform tests. There are documented changes in the H-reflex, a spinal postural reflex mediated by the vestibulo-spinal tract.

All of the above phenomena combine to produce Earth sickness in some small number of people upon return from orbit. From experiences with sailors, it is not unexpected that some would show motion sickness when they return from space.

LONG-TERM EFFECTS

The long-term effects of microgravity on the vestibular system and the central nervous system are not yet known. Although the Soviets have had several long-duration manned flights (up to 237 days), there is very little information published about any long-term vestibular effects from this exposure to microgravity. Several rodent experiments have been performed on the morphological effects of microgravity on the vestibular system and the data are difficult to interpret. It appears that there is a large variation in the size and distribution of the otoconia (small calcium carbonate crystals that are the sensing mechanisms for the otoliths) with respect to earth-bound control animals.

First, the effect of this variability on the response of the otolith system to linear accelerations must be investigated, and second, the Central Nervous System (CNS) interpretation of these possibly different vestibular signals must be studied.

Although the nervous system shows "plasticity"; that is, it can adapt to many different environments, the possibility exists that for multiple generations of animals that are born and bred in space, the CNS might be unable to adapt to return to a normal 1 g environment on Earth. Studies of "functional blindness" caused by sensory deprivation to a kitten's brain indicate that during early development, the CNS is very dependent on a continued, vigorous stimulation of sensory areas. Therefore, these responses to long-term microgravity need to be investigated and can be done only on the Space Station.

IMPLICATIONS FOR FUTURE BIOMEDICAL SUPPORT OF SPACE FLIGHT

Short-Term Effects

The true nature of motion sickness susceptibility in space must be more systematically studied. Because people tend to restrain head motions if they are sick in space, it is important that some standardized test be carried out in the early days of microgravity on crewmembers that are non-essential to orbiter system tasks. These tests are required to better document the true susceptibility to space motion sickness as well as the time course of the adaptation to microgravity. For the Space Station era, space motion sickness will influence only a short portion of the entire mission (3 to 4 days out of 90); yet because the shuttle will be the primary vehicle used to do early construction and possibly carry out scientific research experiments in the short term, the problem needs to be better understood and hopefully solved.

The sensations that occur on reentry need to be better studied and characterized. This will also require non-essential but trained crewmembers to perform experiments to quantify the reentry phenomena. These could be done in the mid-deck with small instruments to avoid problems with landing loads, emergency egress capabilities, etc. It is clear that no person who has spent 90 days on the Space Station should be involved in the flying of the space shuttle, but how do we assure that they can properly accomplish emergency procedures if required?

Long-Term Effects

To extend the human capability in space to periods of time approaching a Mars mission will require experiments in many disciplines. In the vestibular field, it is important to understand the long-term effects of microgravity on the development and maintenance of the otoconia because they are made of calcium carbonate and the entire calcium regulation mechanism response to microgravity is not well understood. Many of these experiments will require animal models so that histological studies and long-term exposure studies can be done. In order to support these studies it is important to begin now to plan for and provide for the facilities needed on the Space Station.

There is not yet enough data on the long-term effects of microgravity on systems like the cardio-vascular system and the musculo-skeletal system to make a decision about artificial gravity needs for a long-term mission. If these systems require some form of artificial gravity, this will be accomplished by rotating the spacecraft. This rotation will continuously stimulate the semicircular canals and also provide inputs to the otoliths. Although some work has been done in slow rotating rooms on the ground, the ability to tolerate sustained rotations in space without getting sick needs to be investigated. Because people will be continuously moving around in the spacecraft as well as moving toward the center and thus reducing the "gravity" level, the extension of the ground studies to space flight will need to be done.

The Skylab experiments in the early 1970's indicated that people were not susceptible to head motions carried out on a rotating chair after six days in space. However, in this case, the rotation was near the center of mass and thus no net acceleration vector was applied. Transferring this information to the situation where people have a combination of a steady-state linear acceleration vector and a changing rotation vector is not trivial.

CONCLUSION

In conclusion, the effects of microgravity on the vestibular system are just beginning to be established. So far most experiments have dealt with the short-term effects of space motion sickness and return-to-Earth phenomena. These will always be important as the space shuttle will be the primary mode of transportation for people to and from orbit even when the Space Station is in operation. Therefore, it is important to search for answers to the problems created by changes in the vestibular system output and central nervous system interpretation.

In the long term, it will be important to investigate the more basic structural changes in the otoconia and also CNS adaptation (is it reversible or not?). The issue of artificial gravity is an important one and needs to be investigated if we are serious about long-duration missions to other planets. While this might be needed as a solution to bone demineralization and cardio-vascular deconditioning, it could provide an undesirable side effect to the vestibular system in the form of either constant or intermittent motion sickness as people move about in a rotating environment.

REDUCED GRAVITY:
A NEW BIOMEDICAL RESEARCH ENVIRONMENT

Robert S. Snyder[*]

Sufficient experiments have now been done inside orbiting spacecraft, such as the Space Shuttle, to confirm that operational parameters and material properties can be quite different in the reduced gravity of space. The principal advantages are the reduced buoyancy-induced fluid convection and sedimentation during the experiment and the disadvantages include the limited access to space for laboratory type research. However, the microgravity environment is a resource that cannot be duplicated on Earth and it will soon become increasingly available on the Space Shuttle and Space Station.

To illustrate the utility of the research capability, experiment programs will be described for continuous flow electrophoresis and protein crystal growth. Continuous flow electrophoresis generated interest several years ago as a separation technique for biological cells and it has problems of operation and apparatus design that are caused by buoyancy-induced convection and sedimentation. A series of electrophoresis experiments were carried out on the Apollo and Space Shuttle to evaluate the important physical effects that influenced the process.

Recently, protein crystal growth in space has drawn significant attention because of the potential applications for determining the three-dimensional structure of the proteins. Theoretical and experimental research indicates that density-driven convective flow patterns at the crystal interface and sedimentation of the crystals during their week-long growth yield small crystals of poor quality. Protein crystals are extremely fragile since they are stabilized by relatively weak crystalline interactions. Therefore, it might be expected that protein crystal formation would be especially affected by fluctuations in the growth environment, including those caused by sedimentation or convection in gravitational fields.

The advantages projected for these and other space research programs are significant and the early results are promising. There are also new ideas that need to be developed as access to space increases.

INTRODUCTION

A large number of experiments investigating materials properties and life sciences are now being proposed for the reduced gravity environment of an orbiting spacecraft, or "microgravity." Actually, a spacecraft orbiting at an altitude of 400 km is only 6 percent farther from the center of the Earth than it would be if it were on

* Biophysics Branch, Space Science Laboratory, Marshall Space Flight Center, Mail Code E976, Huntsville, Alabama 35812.

Earth's surface and the gravitational attraction at that altitude is only 12 percent less. Thus the spacecraft and all its contents are very much under the influence of Earth's gravity and the phenomenon of weightlessness occurs because the spacecraft and its contents are in a state of free fall.

The difference between an orbiting vehicle continuously falling toward the center of the Earth and an object dropped from a great height is that the orbiting vehicle is given an initial velocity such that is trajectory carries it beyond the surface of the Earth before the gravitational acceleration can pull it to the ground. Since the spacecraft and every object in it are being accelerated at the same rate toward the center of the Earth, they fall at the same speed. Since the interior objects tend to remain motionless relative to one another and to the vehicle, they are said to be in a weightless environment. Although the vehicle and all its contents are very much under the influence of gravity, they are only weightless relative to the reference frame moving with the vehicle.

A weightless environment is an ideal situation that, in practice, can never be completely realized in an orbiting spacecraft. There are a number of kinetic effects associated with an actual spacecraft that produce artificial gravity-like forces. Any unconstrained object in a spacecraft is actually in its own orbit around the Earth. Only if an object is located at the center of mass of the spacecraft will it have exactly the same orbit as the vehicle. If an object is released motionless relative to the spacecraft at some distance from the center of mass along the flight path it will have its own orbit relative to that of the spacecraft. These orbits can be circular or elliptical depending on the relative location of object and orientation of the spacecraft. These orbits cause the object to slowly drift away from its initial position as the spacecraft moves around the Earth. The accelerations required to continuously alter the trajectories of such interior objects to keep them in the same relative position are small, on the order of 10^{-7}g (1 ten-millionth of the Earth's gravity) for every meter of lateral displacement from the spacecraft center of mass.

The residual atmosphere even at orbital altitude exerts a slight drag force on the spacecraft and causes a small deceleration of the vehicle. A free object inside the spacecraft is not subject to this force and therefore has an apparent acceleration relative to the spacecraft. At an altitude of 400 km the force imparted to a spacecraft from this drag can be calculated. For the Space Shuttle, this atmospheric drag results in deceleration that is also on the order of 10^{-7}g.

These accelerations represent the quiescent background associated with near-Earth orbital flight. Normal operations within a spacecraft also produce additional accelerations of a random nature which are on the order of 10^{-4} to 10^{-7}g. Accelerations resulting from astronauts' moving from one location to another within the cabin are on the order of 10^{-2} to 10^{-4}g depending on the inertia of the spacecraft and how hard the astronauts push off and stop.

The reduced gravity has a major impact on two physical phenomena, convection and sedimentation. Convection is a flow of liquids or gases due to temperature or density differences between adjacent elements in the fluid. In biological systems, an aqueous fluid expands when heated above 4°C and becomes less dense. In a gravity field, the heated fluid element. Similar convective flows can be produced by compositional differences. Convection is an important method for mixing fluids on Earth and uniformity in space is often diffusion controlled. Thus, advantages in a reduced gravity (restricted convection) can be offset by disadvantages (poor mixing).

Sedimentation or flotation is a problem on Earth when objects of one density (e.g. solid particles, gas bubbles) are desired to be uniformly dispersed in a fluid of a different density. A force proportional to the density difference and the acceleration due to gravity causes the objects to settle or rise and disturbs any intended homogeneous distribution.

The culture of suspended biological cells is an example of the mixed advantages/disadvantages of convection and sedimentation. Since the cells will sediment in most culture fluids, a method must be provided for keeping the cells must also be provided and stirring has apparently satisfied these requirements in the past. In reduced gravity, the cells can remain suspended without external shear forces but all chemical transport will be dominated by diffusion, a very slow process in fluids.

Continuous Flow Electrophoresis

To develop the utility of reduced gravity as a research environment, experiment programs in the laboratory and space have begun in continuous flow electrophoresis. Continuous flow electrophoresis generated interest several years ago as a separation technique for biological cells and it has problems of operation and apparatus design, many of which are gravity related.[1] The selection of the electrophoresis

fluid medium is a compromise between the requirements for viable cells and optimum fractionation. Biological cells prefer immersion in buffered electrolytes of physiological ionic strength. The cells enter the electrophoresis channel at a predetermined concentration in a fluid whose properties are comparable to the flowing curtain buffer medium. The electric field applied to this buffer curtain and sample insertion stream induces an electric current proportional to its electrical conductivity. Cells are typically not very mobile in any electrolyte and high electric fields are required to achieve any significant migration. The combination of high applied voltage and high electrical conductivity results in the generation of intense heat in the fluid medium which can destroy the delicate cells. Fortunately, the mobility of cells increases as the electrophoresis buffer ionic strength is decreased and advantage of this phenomenon can be taken provided cell viability is not affected by the low ion content. A longer residence time in the electrophoresis chamber can also give better separations but cell survival is reduced in low ionic strength buffers even though they are isotonic. This gives a range of options for operation with cells and the buffer medium.

The apparatus design must consider means to remove the heat from the buffer that do not inhibit the separation efficiency. Cooling of the chamber walls is commonly done but this aggravates thermal convection which is proportional to the temperature gradient in the buffer. The thermal convection disrupts the rectilinear flow through the chamber and distorts any separation. Additionally, the temperature gradient causes a gradient in other fluid properties, such as viscosity and electrical conductivity, which further influences flow and particle migration. By making the chambers very thin, gradients in fluid properties and unwanted flows can be minimized, but with a concomitant loss in its efficiency as a preparative electrophoresis device. The chamber cannot be too thin or the sample stream through the chamber will not contain enough cells to permit adequate throughput in a reasonable length of time. The cross-section of the sample stream should be small both in the direction of the electric field to increase the resolution of separation and perpendicular to the field to reduce the impact of the fluid cross flow (electroosmosis) near the walls of the chamber. If the sample stream cross-section is a significant fraction of the chamber thickness, then electroosmotic cross flow is necessary to compensate for the parabilic (Poiseuille) downflow through the chamber and yield at least one relatively narrow fraction. The various interacting phenomena described so far lead to operating procedures and apparatus design that must be a compromise. Since gravity has a role in most of these interactions, reduced gravity can be anticipated to offer some advantages.

A series of electrophoresis experiments on Apollo (1971)[2], Apollo Soyuz Test Project (1975)[3], and Space Shuttle (1983)[4] were carried out in space to show that disturbances due to buoyancy-induced thermal convection and sample sedimentation during the separation process are negligible in reduced gravity. The experiments to date have been small-scale demonstrations of specific principles that have increased our knowledge of electrokinetic and fluid dynamic phenomena and have supported our long range electrophoresis goal to conduct high-resolution purification of biological cells and proteins. At the same time, the limitations of ground-based electrophoretic separators have been documented and new concepts have been proposed for future experiments.

Several laboratory instruments have been constructed utilizing past developments in the design and operation of continuous flow electrophoretic separators by Strickler and Hannig combined with innovative developments in the field of fluids analysis by Saville and Ostrach. Building on these developments the McDonnell Douglas Astronautics Co. (MDAC) designed a continuous flow electrophoresis system that evolved from a detailed survey of the requirements for fractionation of biological materials.

In 1978, MDAC began discussions with NASA on the opportunities to develop a space Continuous Flow Electrophoresis System (CFES) that would incorporate specific modifications to their laboratory instruments to take advantage of weightlessness. The first MDAC flight experiments with the CFES on STS-4 in June 1982 fractionated a proprietary tissue culture medium and evaluated the effect of sample concentration using mixtures of rat and egg albumin. MDAC concluded that there was no loss of resolution at the higher concentrations processed in space. In addition, MDAC reported that the quantity of albumin that could be fractionated in the CFES in space was significantly higher than the quantity that could be processed in their ground laboratory instrument during the same time interval. They proposed that these improvements originated from both instrument modifications and increased sample concentrations permitted by weightlessness. The Ortho Diagnostic

Division of Johnson and Johnson joined with MDAC to separate a sufficient quantity of erythropoeitin for laboratory tests.

Under the terms of the JEA, NASA was provided an opportunity to process two samples on STS-6 in April 1983 and STS-7 in June 1983. All experiment objectives and operational parameters, such as applied field, sample residence time in the field, and buffer composition had to accommodate the MDAC capabilities and NASA flight constraints. The NASA objectives were formulated so as to include validation of the sample concentration effects reported by MDAC on STS-4. The specific objectives were (1) to use a model sample material at a high concentration to evaluate the continuous flow electrophoresis process in the MDAC CFES instrument and compare its separation resolution and sample throughput with related devices on Earth and (2) to expand our basic knowledge of the limitations imposed by fluid flows and particle concentration effects on the electrophoresis process by careful design and evaluation of the space experiment. Hemoglobin and a polysacharide were selected as primary samples for STS-6 and a polystyrene latex particles were chosen for separation on STS-7. These experiments worked well and provided extensive data that is still being analyzed. Reflight of CFES is planned and a series of experiments have been proposed to continue the space research.

Protein Crystal Growth

Recently, protein crystal growth in space has drawn significant attention because of the potential applications for determining the three-dimensional structure of the molecule. Theoretical and experimental research indicates that density-driven convective flow patterns and sedimentation due to gravity can influence crystal growth. As part of a program to investigate the influence of gravity on protein crystal growth, ground- and Shuttle-based experiments are in progress and suitable techniques and equipment for protein crystal growth in space are being developed. The research program includes several phases of hardware development, beginning with a simple prototype system and evolving to an automated protein crystal growth unit that will permit the major variables in protein crystallization to be monitored and controlled during the crystal growth processes. As part of the first step in hardware development, protein crystal growth experiments have been performed on four Shuttle flight missions.[6]

Protein crystals are extremely fragile since they are stabilized by relatively weak crystalline interactions. Therefore, it might be expected that protein crystal formation would be especially affected by fluctuations in the growth environment, including those caused by sedimentation or convection in gravitational fields. Several laboratories around the world are involved in efforts to investigate gravitational effects on protein crystal growth.

The first reported space experiments on Spacelab 1 indicated that space-grown protein crystals are considerably larger than crystals of these proteins obtained under the same experimental conditions on Earth. The results of the four recent Shuttle flights confirm additional advantages to protein crystal growth in space. In microgravity, it is expected that crystals will grow in isotropic environments completely surrounded by the growth medium. Growth in such isotropic environments should affect crystal morphology. Convection in solution growth is caused by density gradients that occur when solute is depleted from the solution at the growing crystal surfaces. Convection will force solution to flow past the crystal, thus bringing material to growing crystal surfaces at a rate that is significantly different from the steady-state diffusion rates that would be predominant in quiescent solutions. The flow patterns may generate significant variations in concentration at different parts of a crystal, thus leading to non-uniform growth rates. Also, convection may lead to significant physical stirring of growth solutions. In general, it is expected that such stirring effects might alter nucleation and growth processes. Contacts with vessel walls can lead to heterogeneous nucleation. In the absence of gravity, it is possible to form stable spherical droplets of crystallizing materials, without the extensive wall effects that generally accompany crystallization experiments on Earth.

The Shuttle experiments were designed to optimize the major variables in vapor diffusion protein crystal growth. Experiments related to drop stability established that in orbit large droplets (30 to 40 microliters) are stable on blunt syringe tips even when Shuttle maneuvering rockets were fired. Although protein crystals have been grown in droplets as large as 80 microliters, the experiments to date indicate that smaller droplets will ensure complete equilibration during the limited period (3 to 7 days) available for protein crystal growth on Space Shuttle missions. Ground-based and flight experiments also have provided qualitative information about equilibration rates within the vapor diffusion chambers. These studies have suggested that equilibration rates are significantly slower under microgravity conditions, presumably because of suppressed convection effects. The vapor equilibration chambers have been designed to accelerate these rates by increasing the surface area of wick exposed in the chambers and decreasing the distance between the protein drop and the wicking material.

During the most recent Shuttle experiments in January 1987 on STS-61C[7], crystals were grown of all proteins that were tested, including hens egg white lysozyme, human serum albumin, human C-reactive protein, bacterial purine nucleoside phosphorylase, canavalin, and concanavalin B. That particular Shuttle mission was prematurely shortened, and the protein crystal growth experiments were deactivated during the third day of the flight. Although many of the protein solutions had not completely equilibrated during that period of time, relatively large x-ray quality crystals were obtained for all of the proteins except lysozyme. In addition, photographic records of the crystallization solutions in the vapor diffusion apparatus were obtained while in orbit.

It appears that the elimination of density-driven sedimentation can affect crystal morphology. The best example of this is canavalin, which in space grew crystals that were dispersed through the droplets. Nearly all the space-grown canavalin crystals appear to have formed from separate nucleation sites, resulting in uniform morphologies. On the other hand, canavalin crystals grown by this method on Earth generally form as fused aggregates at the bottom of the droplets.

An entirely new crystal from which had not previously been identified in ground-based crystal growth experiments was obtained from Shuttle experiments. Crystallization of C-reactive protein has been studied extensively over the past 8 years at the University of Alabama in Birmingham, and only one crystal form has been obtained in these experiments. A new crystal from was first observed for C-reactive protein from experiments on STS-61B, and copious quantities of this crystal form were obtained on STS-61C. It diffracts to an appreciably higher resolution than the original crystal form. The new crystal form has now been obtained in ground-based experiments using the Shuttle hardware, so it may be influenced by altered equilibration rates or other experimental conditions that are hardware-dependent. It is not yet clear how microgravity affects the distribution of these two crystal forms of human C-reactive protein.

It is also not clear whether the internal order or diffraction resolution of space-grown protein crystals are significantly different from those of crystals grown n Earth. It will be necessary to do detailed comparisons involving large numbers of crystals grown under well-controlled conditions on Earth and in space before the potential effects of microgravity on protein crystal quality can be evaluated. However, the early experiments are promising and reflights of the Space Shuttle are anticipated to continue this active research area.

REFERENCES

1. Snyder, R.S., "Separation Techniques," in *Material Sciences in Space - A Contribution on the Scientific Basis of Space Processing,* eds., B. Feuerbacher, H. Hamacher, and R.J. Naumann (Springer-Verlag: Berlin), pp465-481, (1986).

2. Snyder, R.S., R.N. Griffin, A.J. Johnson, H. Leidheiser, Jr., F.J. Micale, S. Ross, C.J. van Oss, and M. Bier, "Free Fluid Electrophoresis on Apollo 16," *Sep. and Purif. Meth., 2*(2), pp259-282, (1973).

3. Allen, R.E., Ph.H. Rhodes, R.S. Snyder, G.H. Barlow, M. Bier, P.E. Bigazzi, C.J. van Oss, R.J. Knox, G.V.F. Seaman, F.J. Micale, and J.W. Vanderhoff, "Column Electrophoresis on the Apollo-Soyuz Test Project," *Sep. and Purif. Meth., 6*(1), pp1-59, (1977).

4. Snyder, R.S., P.H. Rhodes, B.J. Herren, T.Y. Miller, G.V.F. Seaman, P. Todd, M.E. Kunze, and B.E. Sarnoff, "Analysis of Free Zone Electrophoresis of Fixed Erythrocytes Performed in Microgravity," *Electrophoresis, 6*, pp3-9, (1985).

5. Snyder, R.S. et al., "Unexpected Electrophoretic Behavior of Macromolecular Sample on Space Shuttle Flight STS-6," in preparation, (1987).

6. Bugg, C.E., "The Future of Protein Crystal Growth," *J. of Cryst. Growth, 76*, pp535-544, (1986).

7. DeLucas, L.J., F.L. Suddath, R.S. Snyder, R.J. Naumann, M.B. Broom, M.L. Pusey, V. Yost, B.J. Herren, D.C. Carter, B. Nelson, E.J. Meehan, A. McPherson, and C.E. Bugg, "Preliminary Investigations of Protein Crystal Growth Using the Space Shuttle," *J. of Crys. Gro., 76,* pp681-693, (1986).

SOME MEDICAL ASPECTS OF THE SPACE PHOENIX PROGRAM[*]

Thomas F. Rogers[†]

The most fundamental present considerations relative to our having people and things orbiting in the Earth's space are:

a) Other than orbital constraints, the near absence of the influence of the Earth's gravity on activities there

b) The opportunity thereby to obtain, and in some circumstances to use, new physical, psychological and political perspectives

c) The enormous cost of travelling to and from space and of being able to remain there, over time, in a safe and effective fashion.

It is consideration of these enormous costs that form the basis for the following observations. To put them into easily appreciated perspective:

a) It now costs at least some $5,000 per pound to launch anything into Low Earth Orbit (LEO) using Expendable Launch Vehicles (ELVs) and, when the Shuttle fleet begins to operate again, it will cost some $5 million to use it to transport a person on a week's trip to and from LEO.

b) Keeping a 100 watt light bulb lit in LEO for a year costs some $100,000.

c) Extrapolating from the expected cost of the Government's Space Station habitable central complex, a 10' x 10' x 10' "office" in LEO could be expected to cost some $100,000 per day.

Consideration of these, and other related costs, suggests that, for the predictable future, keeping a man or woman in LEO will cost some $100 million a year.

For as long as they obtain, such enormous costs will clearly have a near overriding influence on anything that goes on in space -- its character, magnitude and pace. And it probably means that most of these things will have to be carried on by the government and will have to be paid for by the taxpayer.

In brief: unless such costs are reduced, sharply and soon, and unless many more of our people are able to engage in space activities, directly and personally, the

---

[*] For a detailed description of the Space Phoenix Program see the appendix to this volume.

[†] Dr. Rogers is Chairman, The External Tanks Corporation, 7404 Colshire Rd., McLean, Virginia 22102.

United States, perforce, will have to forgo many tangible and intangible opportunities in the Earth's space.

In this general context, a novel, private, civil space program began to be contemplated some five years ago. This program, the Space Phoenix Program, has as its basic goal the opening up of the Earth's space to the general public. The program now has the formal support of a large and growing number of persons who have a great deal of scientific, engineering and administrative experience in the civil space area, and who share the goal of the Program; and it has captured the positive interest of many space-interested leaders in the Executive and Legislative Branches of the Federal Government.

The Space Phoenix Program's initial approach to cost containment involves making additional long-term in-space use of the large pressure vessel External Tanks (ETs) of the Shuttle fleet. Every ET is now discarded just short of reaching orbit after supplying fuel to an Orbiter's main engines during its ascent to LEO. Using ETs in this fashion avoids a cost of some $300 million per tank for its acquisition cost and transport to LEO. Private resources, including financing, will be employed to modify, outfit and staff the resulting in-orbit habitable facilities. There will be no net out-of-pocket cost to the government. These ET space facilities should be able to be made available at a relatively modest lease price.

The Space Phoenix Program's first objective in the use of such ETs is to see the world's first private in-space scientific research laboratory created and made available to the space-interested science community. This "Labitat" will be used by university and corporation scientists in the conduct of experiments in the life sciences, materials sciences, astronomy, remote sensing, etc.

The accompanying Information Document of the University Corporation for Atmospheric Research Foundation describes the Space Phoenix Program in some detail.

The presence in LEO of a large (at least 70,000 cubic feet) initial habitable facility, staffed by scientists, technicians and operating crew, clearly has important medical connotations:

   a) On a reciprocal basis, it could act as a "safe haven" for the men and women residing at the Government's Space Station.

   b) It could provide support for a wide variety of life science experiments of interest to the space-medical community and to the field of medicine generally.

   c) It could provide a particularly efficient network of life and medical research professionals drawn from the faculties of the 55 University members of UCAR who would be working with the in-space "Labitat" and its scientific research program, and with each other.

   d) It could provide a market for innovative in-space medical equipment and services to be used to support the resident professionals and crews in the Space Phoenix laboratory facility.

Anyone with important space-related medical interests should be informed about the Space Phoenix Program. It is a particularly open-ended program -- one that is designed to encourage university, government, and company scientists and other professionals, to join with it in such a fashion as will serve their professional and business interests and, thereby, the nation's interests in the civil space area.

Note Added in Proof

It is clear from the very informative paper, "Health Maintenance in Orbit", presented here by James S. Logan, M.D. M.S., that the confidence with which Space Station operations could be undertaken would be enhanced greatly if this government facility could have available to it in space, the equivalent of a surface-based, medical-surgical-hospital capability of the type associated with the provision of a first-class, private emergency medical service here on Earth.

Our private medical community should be encouraged by his observations to give early and imaginative consideration to employing basic in-space facilities that could be provided to it by the Space Phoenix Program to assist in the creation of an in-space emergency medical service that would be made available to the government. For not only would the likely morbidity and mortality expectations, otherwise faced by the Space Station's human occupants, be greatly improved thereby but, in the nature of things, the government should be able to obtain such services from the private sector at a lower cost than if it were to set out to provide them itself. Too, the government could avoid appropriating some or all of the large initial capital cost for the Space Station's Health Maintenance Facility (HMF), described by Dr. Logan, (now estimated to cost some $50 million when installed in space) and several hundreds of cubic feet of very valuable Space Station habitable volume would thereby be freed up for other Space Station program purposes. And, in principle as well, having such a facility and service could avoid the truly enormous government capital cost (at least $1 billion) of any Crew Emergency Rescue Vehicle (CERF) and its ongoing O and M costs.

In brief: there would appear to be a fine opportunity for our private medical community to work in cooperation with both the Space Phoenix Program and the Federal Government, especially NASA, so as to provide a first-class, private, in-space emergency medical service at the lowest possible cost and, thereby, decrease morbidity and mortality risks to the Space Station's in-orbit personnel, increase the Space Station's useful volume and avoid the government's need for very large appropriations, including those for any personnel emergency rescue capability.

AAS 87-156

BONE AND MUSCLE MAINTENANCE IN LONG-TERM SPACE FLIGHT, WITH COMMENTARY ON THE AGING PROCESS

Stanley R. Mohler[*]

INTRODUCTION

The genetic plan for skeletal muscle and bone of large mammals is markedly modulated by the applied forces of daily activities. An early student of this topic was Thompson, who pointed out the proportional differences between elephants, humans and mice, based on the interplay between genetic effects and proportional gravitational accelerations (12). He stated: "Man is ruled by gravitation, and rests on Mother Earth". He also observed that "Gravitation influences both our bodies and our mind". In this latter respect he included our knowledge of "up and down" and our architecture of three-dimensional space. Another observer scientist, Julius Wolff, annunciated "Wolff's Law", which states that bone structure and strength develop in opposition to applied forces (15). Land animals have evolved in a gravitational field which provides a continuous force on the skeleton, postural and other working muscles. Additional forces are imposed on the musculoskeletal system based on the types of daily activities and exercises undertaken. For example, today's understanding of the implications of applied forces in athletics is leading to a superior development of muscle and bone elements in athletes, exceeding greatly, no doubt, those of the Greek Olympic period.

As early as 1962, projected similarities between forecast space flight changes during weightlessness and changes associated with advanced age were assessed, the latter derived from the extensive data assembled at the National Institutes of Health (5). A follow-up review of the topic was published in 1985, including the need to stress the tarsal bones during long-term space flight to assume adequate strength on return to one G (6).

In the above connection, it is now clear that skeletal muscle development and maintenance cannot be separated from bone development and maintenance (13). It is also clear that tendons, ligaments and joint development and maintenance, cannot be separated from either skeletal muscle or skeletal bone maintenance. Accordingly, deterioration of skeletal muscles is invariably accompanied by deterioration of associated bone. The same is true in the reverse direction and the same is true with

* Professor and Vice Chair, Department of Community Medicine, Director, Aerospace Medicine, Wright State University, School of Medicine, P.O. Box 927, Dayton, Ohio 45401-0927.

joint morphology and physiology, In view of the foregoing, current evidence demonstrates that, as soon as humans enter the microgravity environment, forces on the spine and other weight-bearing skeletal elements decrease to the point that loss of bone matrix begins almost immediately (7). The muscular effort required to move about within the spacecraft is similarly much less. Associated with these diminished demands upon the non-exercising individual is a loss of intracellular skeletal muscle contractile elements. The body responds in an adaptive fashion to lowered physical demand and, during microgravity, simply produces a physiological adaptation to the "unloaded" environment, that is, diminished muscle mass and loss of calcium from bones.

The most extensive microgravity scientific studies of calcium balance and muscle maintenance were conducted during Skylab 2, Skylab 3 and Skylab 4. The crew and chronology of each are shown in Figure 1. The information in the following sections is a digest of the Skylab findings (3,4,9).

Bone Homeostasis

The daily dietary intake of an astronaut on Skylab 3 (a 59-day mission) is shown in Figure 2 (14). Calcium intake averaged 729 grams per day during flight, a number very close to the preflight level and also the postflight level (especially when the standard deviation is taken into consideration) (14). For the first four shuttle flights, the mean daily calcium consumption was 1210, 687, 885, and 954 milligrams, respectively (10). The NASA-recommended daily allowance (as well as that of the National Academy of Sciences) is 800 milligrams (10). A recent study recommends a daily calcium intake of 1200-1500 milligrams while in microgravity (1). Figure 3 shows the calcium loss that occurred (through urine and feces) in all three Skylab flights (8). The changes in calcium loss during microgravity parallel those seen in bedrest studies (8). The total calcium loss that occurred during the second month in space approximated four grams per month, or about 0.4 percent of the total body calcium per month (8). The calcium loss continued through the third month during Skylab 4. The studies indicate that the loss will most likely continue for a very long time unless protective measures are developed and followed. The studies also project that "thin trabeculae in bone can be returned to normal thickness" upon returning to Earth or arising from prolonged bedrest, but it may be that if the trabeculae are completely lost, they cannot be later restored (8).

Muscle Degeneration

The postural muscles begin to decondition as soon as a microgravity environment is entered (13). The condition of these and other skeletal muscles is directly related to the nature of the physical workloads imposed upon them (13). In Skylab 2, only the bicycle ergometer was used for in-flight exercise, while on Skylab 3, the MK-I (an isokinetic centrifugal brake device) and the MK-II (handles with extension springs) were used as well as the bicycle ergometer, and on Skylab 4, a teflon treadmill was used in addition to the bicycle ergometer and MK-I and MK-II (13).

FIGURE ONE

Skylab	Crew	Dates
TWO:	Conrad (Commander) Kerwin (Scientist Pilot) Weitz (Pilot)	May 25 – June 22, 1973 (28 days)
THREE:	Bean (Commander) Garriott (Scientist Pilot) Lousma (Pilot)	July 28 – September 25, 1973 (59 days)
FOUR:	Carr (Commander) Gibson (Scientist Pilot) Pogue (Pilot)	November 16, 1973 – February 8, 1974 (84 days)

After Johnston and Dietlein

Mean Daily Dietary Intake Commander, Skylab Three (59 day)

	Preflight	Flight	Postflight
Kcal	2,732.0 (113)	2,781.0 (259)	2,940.0 (149)
Protein, g	95.0 (5)	85.0 (11)	96.0 (6)
Nitrogen, g	15.2 (0.9)	13.6 (1.17)	15.4 (1.0)
Potassium, mg	1,517.0 (57)	1,431.0 (116)	1,537.0 (68)
Calcium, mg	725.0 (31)	729.0 (72)	742.0 (40)

(Standard deviation, plus and minus, in parentheses)

After Whedon, et al.

FIGURE THREE

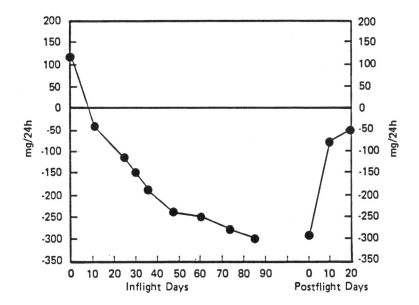

Daily calcium balance changes as Skylab flight duration
increased. By the 84th day of flight, 300 mg. per day
of calcium was lost in the urine and feces.

After Rambaut and Johnston

33

During Skylab 2, the leg muscle extensor strength fell by 25 percent as the bicycle ergometer was insufficiently duplicative of walking forces (13). Arm extensor muscles could be better maintained than were the legs, using the bicycle ergometer by hand. Skylab 3 use of the MK-I and MK-II demonstrated that arm strength could be maintained by devices, but the leg muscle strength was not (13). On Skylab 4, the prior devices were used as well as the treadmill (it weighed 3.5 pounds). The treadmill (which had elastic supports holding the user upon it) was walked upon for about 10 minutes each day, with interspersed jumping and jogging (Note: the elastic cords holding the user to the treadmill placed tension through the tarsal bones, an important consideration in their maintenance as earlier cited). There was only a six percent loss of leg strength during Skylab 4, and post-flight recovery was more rapid than in Skylabs 2 and 3 (see Figure 4). It is concluded that muscle in space is no different from muscle on Earth - proper nourishment and exercise will maintain the strength and function of skeletal muscles (13).

Gaps and Next Steps

The optimal types of muscle and associated bone and exercise levels for maintaining astronauts for return to a one G environment will of necessity be related to the nature and duration of the flight mission, the availability of access to "artificial gravity levels", and future research findings on various mission segment physiologic demands (including extravehicular activities). The need for metabolic energy expenditure data during microgravity activities is pressing. P. Webb and S. Mohler intend to collect data on one aspect of this, specifically determining energy output in space by direct calorimetry utilizing Webb's non-interfering body-suit calorimeter (proposal 284006).

The reversal of the negative calcium balance experienced during microgravity is another priority study that relates to the crews of long-term interplanetary missions (for example, to Mars). A potentially promising avenue of study is the use of anabolic steroids to promote osteogenesis and inhibit bone resorption (11). The information derived from bedrest studies, Soviet long-term flights and Soviet bedrest studies, should provide a significant increment to the base-line countermeasure knowledge currently available. There is reason for guarded optimism that the solutions to muscle and bone maintenance during long-term space flight are within grasp. A suggested approach to providing daily exercise is to provide specific leg muscle stimulation through external skin electrodes (2). In this fashion, the muscles would be maintained without the need for mental concentration on the exercise, freeing the mind for other tasks during the period. These, and other countermeasures to microgravitational changes in bone and muscle are being considered for study on future space flights.

Leg strength loss (crew averages) was only 8 percent during the 84 day flight, a testimony to the benefits of increased exercise.

After Thornton and Rummel

REFERENCES

1. Altman, P.L. and Talbot, J.M., 1987. Nutrition and Metabolism in Spaceflight. *Journal of Nutrition*, March, pp421-427.

2. Buchanan, P., Flores, J.F., Frey, M.A.B., and Duvoisin, M., 1987. Electrical Stimulation to Leg Muscles in Ambulatory Subjects. *Aviation, Space and Environmental Medicine*, May, p500.

3. Johnston, R.S. and Dietlein, L.F., eds., 1977. Biomedical Results from Skylab. NASA Publication SP-377, Washington, D.C., pp1-491.

4. Leach, C.S., Johnson, P.C., Rambaut, P.C., 1976. Metabolic and Endocrine Studies: The Second Manned Skylab Mission. *Aviation, Space, and Environmental Medicine*, 47, pp402-410.

5. Mohler, S.R., 1962. Aging and Space Travel. *Aerospace Medicine*, May, pp594-597.

6. Mohler, S.R., 1985. Age and Space Flight. *Aviation, Space and Environmental Medicine*, July, pp714-717.

7. Nicogossian, E. and Parker, J.F., 1982. Space Physiology and Medicine. NASA Publication SP-447. Washington, D.C., pp1-324.

8. Rambaut, P.C. and Johnston, R.S., 1979. Prolonged Weightlessness and Calcium Loss in Man. *Acta Astronautica.*, 6, pp1113-1122.

9. Rambaut, P.C. and Goode, A.W., 1985. Skeletal Changes During Space Flight. *The Lancet,* November 9, pp1050-1052.

10. Saver, R. and Rap, R., 1983. Food and Nutrition. In Shuttle OFT Medical Report: Summary from STS-1, STS-2, STS-3, and STS-4, NASA TM - 58252, Pool, S.L., Johnson, P.C. and Mason, J.A., eds. NASA, Houston, pp53-62.

11. Stepaniak, P.C., Furst, J.J. and Woodard, D., 1986. Anabolic Steroids as a Countermeasure Against Bone Demineralization During Space Flight. *Aviation, Space, and Environmental Medicine*, February, pp174-178.

12. Thompson, D.W., 1915. On Magnitude. Reprinted in *The World of Mathematics*, Volume Two. J.R. Newman, ed., Simon and Schuster, New York, 1956, pp1001-1046.

13. Thornton, W.E. and Rummel, J.A., 1977. Muscular Deconditioning and Its Prevention in Space Flight. Chapter 21 in *Biomedical Results from Skylab*, NASA SP-377 (Johnston, R.S. and Dietlein, L.F., eds.), pp191-197, NASA, Washington, D.C.

14. Whedon, G.D., Lutwak, L., Rambaut, P.C. Whittle, M.W. Smith, M.C., Reid, S., Leach, C., Studler, C.R. and Sanford, D.D., 1977. Mineral and Nitrogen Metabolic Studies, Experiment MO71. Chapter 18 in *Biomedical Results from Skylab*, NASA SP-377 (Johnston, R.S. and Dietlein, L.F., eds.), pp164-174, NASA, Washington, D.C.

15. Wolff, J., 1868. Wolff's Law. Quoted in Shands, A.R., *Handbook of Orthopaedic Surgery.* C.V. Mosby Co., St. Louis, 1952, p76. Also, 1892, Das Gesetz der Transformation der knocken - Hirschold, Berlin.

CARDIOVASCULAR RESPONSES TO MICROGRAVITY: ADAPTATION, MALADJUSTMENT, AND COUNTERMEASURES

F. Andrew Gaffney[*]

Humans have worked in space for up to 237 days without significant in-flight limitations, although major cardiovascular disability is seen following space flight of even a few days duration. Most of the cardiovascular research on microgravity deconditioning has been observational in character. Detailed studies of mechanisms and causes of post-flight exercise intolerance, low blood pressure and fainting in astronauts and cosmonauts have not been done, despite almost 30 years of manned space flight. A review of possible mechanisms of post-flight cardiovascular deconditioning and directions for study is provided.

INTRODUCTION

Prior to the first manned space flight, a number of dire predictions were made regarding the physiological effects of microgravity. Fortunately, fluid-filled lungs, swollen brains, and decreased circulation to the legs were not found. In fact, human space flight experience spanning almost 30 years has not shown any specific adverse cardiovascular effects of living in microgravity. The body seems to adapt rapidly and well when going from Earth's gravity to the microgravity of space. The converse however, is not true, and major physiological problems occur when one re-experiences gravity following weightlessness. This paper reviews the cardiovascular changes known or believed to occur in crew members who must transition from weightlessness to gravity fields. In order to understand these changes, a brief review of the normal physiological responses to gravity will be given.

CARDIOVASCULAR PHYSIOLOGY IN GRAVITY

The major challenge faced by man's cardiovascular system is the maintenance of blood pressure and flow to the brain and other vital organs against the hydrostatic pressure gradient produced by standing. This is accomplished with a complex system of both high- and low-pressure sensors, central and peripheral processors, and effector components.

---

[*] M.D., University of Texas Health Science Center at Dallas; Payload Specialist, Spacelab Life Sciences 1; Currently at NASA Headquarters, Life Sciences Division, 600 Independence Ave., S.W., Mail Code EBM, Washington, D.C. 20546.

The main high-pressure receptors, *carotid baroreceptors*, are strategically located in the neck, and sense both pulsatile and mean pressure levels of blood flowing to the brain. The advantages of locating these sensors so close to the *central computer* are obvious. Other high-pressure sensors, located downstream in the aorta, monitor the pressure of blood flowing to the kidneys, intestines, and the lower half of the body. These high-pressure receptors detect changes in arterial pressure and evoke reflex changes in pumping rate (heart rate) and blood vessel resistance (vasoconstriction or vasodilation). By varying both flow rate and resistance, pressure is finely regulated.

The low-pressure receptors are located in the atria of the heart and in the veins which return blood to the heart from the lungs. These receptors provide information about heart chamber volumes. They too regulate arterial blood pressure through reflex constriction or dilation of arteries but, unlike the high-pressure receptors, have little effect on heart rate.

When one stands, gravity causes pooling of blood below the level of the heart, and reduces blood returning to the heart. This, in turn, reduces the quantity of blood which is pumped from the heart. The high-pressure receptors sense the resulting decrease in arterial pressure and the low-pressure receptors detect the decreased heart volume. Concordant signals are received by blood pressure control centers located in the brainstem. Reflex constriction of small arteries increases arterial resistance and acceleration of heart rate augments blood flow and returns pressure to normal or even to slightly supra-normal levels.

This tendency for arterial pressure to rise slightly above normal when one stands is interesting in that one usually considers closed-loop feedback systems capable of partial, but never perfect correction of an error condition. It is the dual input of both pressure and volume signals that allows this over-correction. Pressure may be over-corrected when one stands, but heart volume remains low and arterial resistance remains high.

This dual input of both pressure and volume information may increase the tendency of astronauts to faint while standing quietly after space flight. Heart chamber volumes are extremely low following space flight because of pooling of blood below heart level and a decrease in blood volume produced by space. As the heart pumps more vigorously to maintain flow to the body, the low-pressure receptors are stimulated paradoxically, as though the pressure were too high. This produces slowing of the heart rate and dilation of the arteries. Blood pressure is lowered even further and fainting occurs.

Somewhat surprisingly, the veins play only a minor role in acute postural adjustments. They constrict very little in the first few minutes of standing, but do increase tone after several minutes, probably due to rising blood levels of the vasoconstrictor norepinephrine. The leg muscles also play a significant role in blood pressure regulation through their control of venous volume. The pumping action of the muscles which augments return of venous blood to the heart during exercise is important and well-known. Less well-known is the mechanism by which distension of the leg veins with pooling blood reflexively increases tone in the leg muscles and improves venous return to the heart. Finally, there is augmented carotid pressure receptor sensitivity through signals originating in the gravity sensing vestibular system which is activated by standing. These latter two mechanisms have been shown in animals, but proof in man is not available.

CARDIOVASCULAR PHYSIOLOGY IN MICROGRAVITY

The cardiovascular system faces the reverse problem when adjusting to microgravity. The absence of a downward hydrostatic pressure causes blood which normally pools in the legs and abdomen to remain in the chest, neck and head. The face becomes puffy, there is bothersome nasal congestion, and the legs become skinny (bird legs). About 12% of the total leg volume is lost in the first days of flight,mostly in the first few hours. This corresponds to a headward fluid shift of about 2.5 liters. Presumably, the increase of blood in the chest is sensed by the low-pressure receptors as an excess of volume. An increase in the clearance of salt and water via the kidneys could be expected until the blood volume in the chest returned to normal. Unfortunately, it is not known whether or not any fluid loss occurs by this mechanism.

Several factors have prevented an accurate determination of urine volumes early in flight. In many ways, the problems encountered in accomplishing something as simple as measuring urine volume exemplify the difficulties one faces while doing medical research in space. In all the U.S. flights to date, the headward fluid shift and increased urine flow probably began before launch, while crew members spent several hours on the pad, lying on their backs, with their legs elevated. (The lack of understanding of this simple physiological principle that raising the legs may increase urine output created some major and well-publicized logistical problems early in our space program...) Thus, the headward fluid shifts and accompanying adaptation may occur before the crew ever launches! Another confounding factor is that some crew members dehydrate themselves before flight in the reasonable, but unproven belief that they will avoid the nasal congestion and other symptoms of the headward fluid shifts. Finally, space motion sickness, which produces loss of appetite, nausea and vomiting in up to half of the crew members also causes dehydration. Together, these factors have hidden any increase in urine output if it occurs at all. For all these reasons, the time course, magnitude, and duration of the fluid shifts and adaptation to them are almost completely unknown.

After a few days in space, the cardiovascular system appears to compensate completely and normally for these headward fluid shifts. Blood pressure and heart rate remain normal, relative to pre-flight standing values, although values are higher if compared to the control values measured with the subject lying down. Heart chamber volumes measured by echocardiography inflight rose initially and then decreased to standing pre-flight levels. These data suggest that man's circulatory system is adjusted or set to operate with *standing* as the reference position. This has been the subject of great debate among physiologists in the past and provides evidence that would not be available were it not for space medical research.

Further proof of the complete adjustment 0-g is found in the Skylab date which shows that aerobic exercise capacity, measured in-flight on a stationary bicycle, was maintained. Maximal exercise was not determined on those flights, but will be obtained during the 7-day Spacelab mission SLS-1 scheduled for launch early in 1990. The inflight measurement of maximal exercise capacity after only 5-6 days is useful in that it permits differentiation of changes due to fluid shifts from those due to muscle wasting seen on longer flights. Preservation of inflight exercise capacity despite full cardiovascular adaptation to microgravity would suggest that countermeasures aimed at maintaining capacity on long-duration flights should focus on muscular factors rather than circulatory parameters.

POSSIBLE CARDIOVASCULAR PROBLEMS IN MICROGRAVITY

There have been some questions regarding losses in heart muscle mass during space flight, but there are no data to suggest that this is a problem. Heart muscle mass in normal subjects is closely regulated as a function of the stress imposed on individual muscle fibers by the pressure and diameter of the left ventricle,the main pumping chamber of the heart. Higher pressure or a larger diameter would raise heart wall stress and cause thickening. High blood pressure, heart failure or high levels of fitness are all associated with some thickening. In space, blood pressure remains normal, and heart chamber volumes are reduced to approximately the volume found in a standing person. Thus, heart mass would not be expected to change in space flight.

Some crew members have experienced minor benign irregularities of heart rhythm in flight. These are supposed to be more common during extravehicular activity (EVA), but to a certain extent, this may represent a sampling bias, in that EVA is the only time when U.S. crew members are routinely monitored. The extent of actual arrhythmias is unknown, but should be ascertained. Heart rhythm is easily recorded with widely available equipment, and establishment of a data base would be essential in determining whether there is a potential problem. Perhaps more importantly, a data base could document the insignificance of a serendipitously detected arrhythmia, as is the case for most arrhythmias in healthy subjects on the ground. An adequate data base may have led Soviet physicians to avoid terminating a long-duration flight for *Cardiac Problems* as they did recently.

PROBLEMS ON RETURN TO GRAVITY AFTER SPACE FLIGHT

Whereas space flight is rather benign for the cardiovascular system inflight, the same is not true when returning to a 1-g environment. Many astronauts and cosmonauts suffer profound drops in blood pressure when attempting to stand up in 1-g. The problem of low blood pressure is sufficiently severe that cosmonauts often require several days before blood pressure control is adequate for quiet standing. Shuttle crews returning from flights of only 4-10 days have similar problems, although of lesser magnitude. Five minutes of quiet standing immediately after flight will cause fainting or near fainting in a majority of astronauts. Several explanations for this fall in blood pressure on standing have been suggested.

Blood volume is reduced approximately 1 pint following flight. This is the amount of blood taken in a routine blood donation. The symptoms after flight, however, are much worse than would be expected after donating blood. The administration of salt and water to both Soviet and U.S. crews has improved standing blood pressure levels somewhat, but blood pressure regulation is not normalized entirely. Blood volume is probably not completely restored by taking an arbitrary amount of salt and water before re-entry. The amount of salt water entering the circulation and the time it remains there are important but unkown variables. This has led some investigators to seek other causes of the poor blood pressure control. They have focused on the other mechanisms of blood pressure control described above. A number of these mechanisms will be determined in more detail on an upcoming Spacelab mission.

EXPERIMENTS ON SPACELAB LIFE SCIENCES 1

The first dedicated NASA Life Sciences mission, Spacelab Life Sciences 1, will examine cardiovascular function in detail by comparing pre- and post-flight measurements with those made during the flight itself. The validity of head-down tilt bedrest, the most commonly used models for simulating the fluid shifts seen in microgravity, will also be determined. The crew will participate as subjects in a head-down tilt bedrest study pre-flight. This study and the flight itself will include direct measurement of central venous pressure, obtained by passing a small plastic catheter through an arm vein into the chest. This *filling pressure* is the major determinant of the output of the heart. Heart chamber dimensions will be measured by 2-dimensional echocardiography, a phased-array ultrasound heart imaging system. Cardiac output, the quantity of blood pumped through the heart per minute, is measured by the non-invasive CO_2 rebreathing technique. This method, an indirect Fick technique, estimates the amount of blood passing through the lungs by determining the quantity of CO_2 expired by the subject, and the concentration of CO_2 of the blood in the lungs. A mass spectrometer, high-precision gas flow meter, and a microcomputer are required.

The sensitivity of the high-pressure sensors in the carotid arteries in the neck will be determined by a specially constructed silastic neck cuff which fits snugly over the front of the neck. Pressure or suction in this neck chamber decreases or increases the stretch on the pressure sensors in the neck, and *fools* the cardiovascular regulatory system. The resulting changes in heart rate, faster when the blood pressure is sensed as falling, and slower when the blood pressure seems to rise, are recorded. The relationship between neck cuff pressure and heart rate describes the sensitivity of the sensor system.

Changes in hormones which regulate fluid volume, salt retention, and blood production will be measured several times during the flight. An on-board blood processing kit, clinical centrifuge, and -20 degree C freezer allow investigators to make far more detailed measurements than either the U.S. or the Soviets have been able to make in the past. Radioisotopes will be administered at early, intermediate,

41

and late points in the flight to characterize changes in kidney function and blood and plasma volumes.

THE NEED FOR DEDICATED, INTEGRATED MISSIONS

The integrated approach planned for SLS-1 and SLS-2 scheduled for 1992, represents a major improvement over previous U.S. and Soviet flight experiments which have tended to be anecdotal, with a few measurements being made on different subjects on different flights. The lack of appropriate hardware, small number of observations, changes in protocols, variations in environmental factors, and the natural variability of human physiological data have made careful analysis of mechanisms impossible to date. This lack of understanding of mechanisms has prevented the development of effective countermeasures for short- or long-duration space flights, but their ability to do so quickly in the case of a landing emergency is severely reduced in some cases, and presents a real risk, thus far not solved. Most U.S. airlines would not allow passengers in the debilitated condition of returning astronauts to occupy Exit row seats!

COUNTERMEASURES

The problems following long-duration flights are far more severe, but equally unsolved. The Soviets use a vigorous, time-consuming in-flight exercise program with both a treadmill and an exercise bicycle. The cosmonauts also wear suits with bungee cords to cause tension on the muscles. In the 2-3 weeks prior to re-entry, they also use lower body negative pressure to *re-acclimatize* the veins in the legs. Finally, they give their crews large amounts of salt and water immediately prior to re-entry. Despite this, cosmonauts are generally lifted from their re-entry vehicle on stretchers and are not able to walk well for several days.

THE CHALLENGE

The U.S. program faces major problems in the 1990's, when the Space Station and flights of six months or longer become a reality. The Soviets have established an impressive record of long-duration space flight. They also have a record of consistent victories in Olympic competition demonstrating their expertise in areas such as exercise physiology and muscle mechanics. Nonetheless, cardiovascular deconditioning after long-duration space flight remains a mystery both in terms of causes and treatments. Hopefully, the U.S. will not continue to depend so heavily on the Soviets for their space medicine research. U.S. goals for humans in space, this century and the next, demand better!

GENERAL REFERENCES

1. "Biomedical Results from Skylab," L.F. Dietlein, R.S. Johnston, Eds. *NASA Special Publication* 377, pp 284-407, 1977.

2. C.G. Blomqvist, H.L. Stone, "Cardiovascular Adjustments to Gravitational Stress," in *Handbook of Physiology*. Section 2: The Cardiovascular System, Vol. 3 (J.T. Shepherd, F.M. Abboud, Eds.) Bethesda, MD, American Physiological Society, pp 1025-1063, 1983.

3. C.G. Blomqvist, F.A. Gaffney, J.V. Nixon, "Cardiovascular responses to head-down tilt in young and middle-aged men," *The Physiologist* 26(6):S-81-82, 1983.

4. "Research Opportunities in Cardiovascular Deconditioning," M.N. Levy, J.M. Talbot, Eds., Federation of American Societies for Experimental Biology, Bethesda, MD, 1983, *NASA Contractor Report 3707.*

5. M.W. Bungo, D.J. Goldwater, R.L. Popp, H. Sandler, "Echocardiographic Evaluation of Space Shuttle Crew Members," *J. Appl. Physiol.* 62:278-283, 1987.

6. F.A. Gaffney, "Spacelab life sciences experiments: An integrated approach to the study of cardiovascular deconditioning and orthostatic hypotension," *Acta Astronautica,* 15:291-294, 1987.

7. J.M. Fritsch, D.L. Eckberg, R.L. Goble, J.J. Schelhron, H.C. Halliday, "Device for rapid quantification of human carotid baroreceptor-cardiac reflex responses," *J. Appl. Physiol.,* 60:727-732, 1986.

SOVIET MANNED SPACE FLIGHT:
PROGRESS THROUGH SPACE MEDICINE

Victoria Garshnek[*]

This paper provides an historical overview of the Soviet Space Program, in particular, how space medicine has helped shape the destiny and progress of the Soviet manned space flight effort. Building on past experience and knowledge, Soviet space medicine has become broad, comprehensive, and forward-looking. The Soviet space station program has provided the capability to investigate the long-term influence of microgravity on human physiology and to test various countermeasures against the physiological deconditioning effects of microgravity. In view of the physiological problems that may be encountered during extended space missions, it is critical that certain countermeasures be developed if manned space flights beyond one year are to become a reality. The Soviets are actively pursuing studies to this end. Already a one-year bed rest study incorporating countermeasures (exercise, diet, pharmaceutical) has been completed. Results of such studies, as well as the continued completion of long-duration missions, may provide the necessary knowledge to proceed with greater confidence toward extending human stay time and productivity in space.

HISTORICAL SURVEY: FROM SPUTNIK THROUGH SALYUT

Early Activities

At the turn of the century, Konstantin Tsiolkovsky, a small-town Russian schoolteacher, formulated the theoretical foundations for the Soviet space program with his visionary writings of orbiting manned space stations as springboards to the cosmos. On October 4, 1957, the launch of Sputnik 1 opened the path toward the realization of Tsiolkovsky's dream.

Having demonstrated the ability to orbit functioning hardware, the Soviets launched Sputnik 2 one month later, carrying a dog named Laika. Laika's cabin contained air regeneration and thermal regulation systems, and equipment for monitoring pulse, respiration, blood pressure, and heart activity. Environmental and physiological parameters were telemetered back to Earth throughout the one-week flight (Ref. 1). This historical event ushered in a new era of biomedical research in space and offered the first evidence that a higher vertebrate, fairly similar to man physiologically, could not only withstand the rigors of rocket launch, but could also tolerate, for at least one week, a variety of space flight factors.

---

* Ph.D., The George Washington University, Washington, D.C. 20006.

These endeavors were subsequently extended in a series of five "Korabl Sputnik" flights, culminating in the historic flight of Vostok 1 on April 12, 1961, which carried Yuri Gagarin -- the first human to orbit the Earth. Comprised of six flights, the Vostok series was similar in purpose to the six U.S. Mercury flights: to establish the basic parameters of human reaction to space flight. The final Vostok flight won the Soviets another first: Valentina Tereshkova became the first woman in space.

After the Vostok series, the Soviets made two more launches of the same spacecraft, but renamed Voskhod ("sunrise"). In October, 1964, Voskhod 1 flew the first crew of three. On this particular mission, inclusion of the first physician in space (Yegorov) allowed for more comprehensive medical data to be obtained in flight. The flight also included on-board studies of hearing, lung function, the vestibular apparatus, and muscle strength in weightlessness. In March of 1965, Voskhod 2 was launched with two cosmonauts on board. With the aid of an accordion-like external airlock and wearing a self-contained life support system, Alexsey Leonov completed man's first "space walk." The extravehicular activity (EVA) consisted of 12 minutes outside the spacecraft and 10 minutes in the depressurized, inflatable airlock (Ref. 2).

The Voskhod flights were followed by a period of inactivity by the Soviets. Meanwhile, the U.S. Gemini Program continued, executing rendezvous and docking maneuvers in space, extending the duration of manned space flight, and performing EVA (the next Soviet EVA was not until the 1969 Soyuz 4/5 flight). After this two-year pause, the Soviets embarked in 1967 on the long-running Soyuz ("Union") program of manned space flight. A major objective of this program was to provide a spacecraft which could be used in space station operations: for supply, transport, and as a free flyer conducting additional independent studies of space (Ref. 3). Tragically, during the first trial of this new vehicle, the Soyuz 1 lost attitudinal stability upon reentry; the parachute system failed, resulting in the death of cosmonaut Vladimir Komarov.

In subsequent Soyuz flights (after a delay of 18 months) cosmonauts exercised skills that would later be integrated into Salyut space station operations: rendezvous, docking, and EVA. Medical monitoring of cosmonauts during the Soyuz program focused on assessing the physiological effects of weightlessness. Cardiorespiratory measurements as well as extensive pre- and postflight examinations were made of the central nervous system, metabolism, blood chemistry, and fluid-electrolyte balance (Ref. 1).

From its first flight in April, 1967, to the landing of Soyuz 9 in June, 1970, Soyuz spacecraft flew 15 persons on eight missions for a total of nearly 44 days of operation in space. The success of Soyuz removed most major technological barriers to the Salyut space station program (a major stepping stone toward permanent presence in space). Soyuz, with evolutionary modifications, remains the standard vehicle to this day for transporting crewmembers to the Mir space station.

The early Soyuz program, consisting of short-duration flights, revealed no unusual or unexpected physiological changes. Cosmonauts were carefully monitored to assess the physiological effects of weightlessness and became more involved in biomedical studies. Strong emphasis was placed on such countermeasures against physiological deconditioning as chest expanders, isometric exercises, elastic tension straps, and the "Penguin" suit (which creates constant compression of the leg and torso muscles) (Ref. 4, 5).

First Generation Space Stations: Salyuts 1-5

The early 1970's witnessed the beginning of the Salyut space station series. By then, confidence had increased that humans could tolerate missions of long duration. The Salyut space stations were intended for long-term habitation of rotating crews, complete with extensive on-board systems, scientific equipment, and a power generator. Facilities were provided for maintenance and housekeeping, as well as eating, sleeping, hygiene, and exercise (Ref. 1, 4).

Salyut 1 was placed in orbit on April 19, 1971. The first crew, Soyuz 10, docked but could not enter. However, the second attempt was successful and the three-man Soyuz 11 crew occupied the space station for three weeks, conducting scientific experiments which included biomedical studies of long-duration weightlessness and exercise countermeasures. Tragically, the crew died during reentry, when a faulty valve opened at the instant of explosive separation of the command and orbital modules, allowing the spacecraft atmosphere to escape into space. Crewmembers were not wearing space suits, and the men died of dysbarism. The accident precipitated a lengthy delay during which safety measures were evaluated. Not until September 1973 was another mission, Soyuz 12, flown. The Soviets returned to two-man crews in the Soyuz, so there would be sufficient room for the cosmonauts to wear space suits. Nearly ten years elapsed before they were able to redesign the Soyuz so that three people could once again be accommodated.

While the American Skylab was in orbit, the Soviets began encountering difficulties in their space station program. On the heels of the staggering Soyuz 11 tragedy, the next space station they launched in 1973 failed as soon as it reached orbit. Not until 1974 did the Soviets succeed in placing another station in orbit -- Salyut 3.

Noteworthy modifications in the Salyut 3 configuration included higher efficiency power and life support systems, and a more "homelike" interior design and decoration. The first crew to dock was Soyuz 14, residing on board Salyut 3 for 14 days. During their stay the cosmonauts conducted some 400 scientific and technical experiments. Physical exercises to assess the effect of physical conditioning on readaptation to gravity were again performed. A treadmill and improved Penguin suit were utilized in the exercise routines (Ref. 5, 6). Medical experiments included studies of cerebral blood circulation and a trial blood velocity. In addition, a daily schedule was devised, allowing for 8 hours sleep, 8 hours work, and 8 hours for exercise and administrative/housekeeping duties (Ref. 1, 6). The next crew (Soyuz 15) was unable to dock. Overall, the station remained operational for twice its design lifetime.

In December, 1974, the Soviets launched Salyut 4, which remained in orbit for two years. The first mission to the Salyut 4 space station was Soyuz 17. Again, cosmonauts evaluated various exercise and diet countermeasures against the deconditioning effects of microgravity and studied the cardiovascular system. The "Chibis" vacuum suit (a variant of a lower body negative pressure device(was worn during exercise and for extended periods during normal activity, in an effort to reduce cardiovascular deconditioning and reduce the volume of headward fluid shifts. In addition, a rotating chair similar to that used on Skylab was installed for observing vestibular function. With Soyuz 17, a standard exercise regimen began to emerge: three days of regulated exercise (three times per day, 2.5 hours total) followed by a fourth day on which the selection of exercise was optional. A bicycle ergometer was now included, in addition to the treadmill. Another new approach to physical conditioning was electrical stimulation of various muscle groups by means of the "Tonus" apparatus (Ref. 1).

The Soyuz 17 crew remained in orbit for 29 days. Their successor mission, Soyuz 18A, was aborted during ascent. Next on board the Salyut 4 was the Soyuz 18B team, who remained in orbit for 62 days and continued the research programs. A new cardiovascular countermeasure combined physical exercise with a high-salt diet and forced intake of water to increase body fluid volume. This was done during the final ten days of flight to prepare the cosmonauts for return to gravity.

Salyut 5 was launched June 22, 1976. The Soyuz 21 crew remained in the station for 49 days, and the crew of Soyuz 24 remained on board for 16 days (Soyuz 22 was a free flying mission and the crew of Soyuz 23 failed to dock). Crews again employed forced water and high-salt diet before return to Earth. Salyut 5 was the last in that series to carry only one docking port, a design characteristic that prevented a resupply vehicle from docking when a crew was already onboard (an important consideration for flights of longer duration). This concern led to the development of the "Progress" cargo ship, capable of bringing scientific equipment, food, clothing, water, compressed air, and fuel to the space station. The vehicle could also remove "garbage" by separating from the station and performing a destructive reentry over the ocean.

Second Generation Space Stations: Salyuts 6 and 7

To accommodate the Progress cargo ship or an additional visiting Soyuz crew, a second generation space station, Salyut 6, incorporated an additional docking unit at the opposite end of the station. Salyut 6 was launched September 29, 1977. The station could be refueled in orbit, and included a shower and water-regeneration device supplying crewmembers with wash water (fresh drinking water was stored). Salyut 6 cosmonauts also tested newly designed EVA space suits and routinely worked as orbital repairmen, greatly extending the station's design life of 18 months.

With Salyut 6, great interest centered on further extending the duration of manned flight and determining whether barriers exist to the endurance of weightlessness. Five long-duration "prime" crews (Soyuz 26, 29, 32, 35, T-4) carried out missions lasting 96, 140, 175, 185, and 75 days, respectively. Both for psychological relief and for practice in multimanned station operation, prime crews were periodically visited by 11 other crews, each of which typically stayed for a week. During this period, two crews did not dock (Soyuz 25 and 33) and of the participating cosmonauts, six made two flights to the station, and seven spent more than 100 days in space.

To maximize psychological adaptation to space flight, Soviet medical specialists instituted on Salyut 6 a sleep-wake-work cycle keyed to normal Moscow time, with a 5-day work week and 2-day weekend. A comprehensive psychological support program included frequent communications with families, radio and television programs, and delivery of gifts, letters, news, and favorite foods via the Progress cargo ship. These measures appeared to make the long-term isolation and workload tolerable.

The "Interkosmos" program carried out during this period involved cosmonauts from nine Soviet bloc nations (Bulgaria, Cuba, Czechoslovakia, the German Democratic Republic, Hungary, Mongolia, Poland, Romania, and Viet Nam) as "visiting crewmembers." Biomedical activities focused on acute physiological adaptation through a variety of medical investigations utilizing instruments developed by the participating nations.

The Salyut 6 period also saw the successful flight of a new model of the Soyuz ferry craft, designated Soyuz T. The first manned flight of the new craft, T-2, took place in June, 1980. Soyuz T-3 was a two-week demonstration of its capability to carry a crew of three. The Soyuz T-4 was used to transport the final prime crew to Salyut 6, while two visiting crews (Soyuz 39 and 40) utilized the previous version of Soyuz for the last time.

In addition to the Soyuz-T and Progress vehicles, multiple crew dockings, and refueling in orbit, Salyut 6 operations introduced the Kosmos 1267 module, which docked with the space station in June, 1981. Linked with the Salyut 6, the new spacecraft was tested as a mid-orbital tug. Kosmos 1267 also represented a "prototype space module," intended and constructed to expand future station operations. Such modules would be dedicated to scientific pursuits, or outfitted as living quarters.

Salyut 6 remained on orbit for 4 years and 10 months. After Salyut 7 was launched, Kosmos 1267 propelled Salyut 6 into a destructive reentry on July 29, 1982. The experience of the Salyut 6 crews, particularly on the 6-month missions, gave medical planners and researchers confidence that longer exposures to weightlessness and other flight factors were possible.

Salyut 7 was launched in April, 1982. With two docking ports (one of which had been modified to handle larger spacecraft) this version was similar in size and shape to Salyut 6. Station operations were further automated and recommendations from cosmonauts who had lived on board Salyut 6 led to an interior "modernization program" to make Salyut 7 more livable. Designers took special care to protect certain observation windows, the color scheme was changed to improve the working environment, and a refrigerator was installed (Ref. 7). New systems for medical examination and diagnosis improved the range of biomedical parameters that could be monitored, either on board by the cosmonauts or remotely by ground control.

The Soyuz T-5 transported the first crew to the Salyut in May, 1982. The crew of two performed about 300 experiments and set a new endurance record for space flight: 211 days. A visiting crew of three from Soyuz T-6 included a French "spationaut", Jean-Loup Chretien, who performed cardiovascular studies utilizing the "French Echocardiograph." On a separate occasion, Soyuz T-7 carried another crew of three, including the world's second woman cosmonaut, Svetlana Savitskaya.

A modular transport ship, Kosmos 1443, docked with Salyut 7 on March 10, 1983, in a configuration similar to the Salyut 6/Kosmos-1267 complex. Kosmos 1443 functioned both as an automatic space cargo vehicle (to return materials and research data base to Earth) and as a mid-orbital tug. In April, 1983, Soyuz T-8 failed to dock with the Salyut 7/Kosmos 1443 complex, causing the mission to be aborted. Two months later, the Soyuz T-9 ship, carrying Cosmonauts Lyakhov and Aleksandrov, docked with the scientific research complex, returning to Earth after 150 days in space. The crew carried out scientific experiments during their lengthy flight, including preparation of a pure protein on the Tavriya biotechnological device. In the course of two space walks totaling 5 hours 45 minutes, Lyakhov and Aleksandrov installed additional solar batteries on the station, once again illustrating the skill and confidence of crewmembers to perform extravehicular maintenance. Crew medical checkups were carried out regularly and a set of prophylactic measures helped maintain good health and a high capacity for work and EVA.

An attempt to send a two-man replacement crew in September was aborted by a launch pad explosion, from which the cosmonauts escaped unharmed. However, on February 9, 1984, the crew of the third main expedition, Soyuz T-10, comprised of cosmonauts Kizim, Solovyev, and Atkov (inflight physician) began work onboard the space station. The crew carried out a considerable amount of research. Galactic and cosmic radiation were evaluated and medical studies by Dr. Atkov evaluated the cosmonauts' health, fitness, and work capacity. Ultrasound equipment was used to monitor cardiovascular activity. The "Glyukometr" ("Glucose meter") device enhanced biochemical investigations into the nature of carbohydrate and mineral metabolism after a long period of time under space flight conditions. The "Sport" experiment was conducted to choose an optimum set of physical exercises and increase their effectiveness during space flight. This experiment determined the level of the cosmonauts' work capacity and the state of their cardiovascular and motor systems in relation to the intensity, methods, and techniques of training routines. The entire crew underwent medical tests to evaluate the reaction of the circulatory system to simulated hydrostatic pressure generated with the "Chibis" suit. Studies were also made of the bioelectric activity of the heart at rest (Ref. 8).

The primary crew performed six space walks, lasting a total of 22 hours and 50 minutes, and carried out intricate and demanding assembly operations to install a bypass circuit for the reserve fuel line of the joint propulsion unit and erect two additional solar cell panels. The final (sixth) EVA occurred six months into the flight, demonstrating the capability of cosmonauts to perform significant physical extravehicular work after prolonged weightlessness.

On April 3, 1984, a visiting crew comprised of Myashev, Strekalov, and Sharma (India) were launched to the Salyut 7 in their Soyuz T-11 vehicle. This was the first time six cosmonauts would work together on board the space station. During their stay, the crew completed scientific investigations, including medical research to improve prophylactic techniques and establish an optimum work/rest schedule.

July 17 of the same year saw the launch of Soyuz T-12 carrying another visiting crew: Cosmonauts Dzhanibekov, Savitskaya, and Volk. One outstanding event during their 12-day visit was the space walk of Svetlana Savitskaya, the first by a woman. During the 3 hours and 35 minutes of her EVA she performed a variety of manual tasks (spraying coatings, welding).

The mission of the primary crew was completed on October 2, 1984. The results of the vast array of studies and experiments conducted during the 237-day flight will undoubtedly have broad applications in future manned space stations.

On June 6, 1985, the Soviet Union launched two cosmonauts aboard a Soyuz T-13 spacecraft. Savinykh and Dzhanibekov efficiently carried out a series of difficult repairs and rehabilitation operations on board the station, which had been shut down at the conclusion of the previous 237-day mission. The cosmonauts again continued with investigations of the cardiovascular system in combination with the "Chibis" pneumatic vacuum suit.

Soyuz T-14, with a visiting crew consisting of Vasyutin, Grechko, and Volkov, was launched September 17 to dock with the orbital complex Salyut 7/Soyuz T-13. The five-member crew carried out a series of experiments with a new electrophoresis unit, the "EFU Robot." Dzhanibekov and Grechko returned to Earth in the Soyuz T-13, leaving Savinykh with the new crew to complete the experiments. As with previous crews, the cosmonauts underwent conditioning with the aid of the "Chibis" suit before returning to Earth's gravity on September 26. Vasyutin and Volkov continued their experiments, which included investigating the possibilities of reflex diagnostics in evaluating physical effects of weightlessness. On November 21, the Soviets terminated the flight when Vasyutin became ill and had to be returned to Earth for hospital treatment. This termination due to illness was another "first" for the Soviets in space, albeit an unfortunate one.

With the return of Savinykh, Vasyutin, and Volkov, the "Salyut era" was essentially completed. The Salyut program contributed considerable information concerning the ability of humans to function for long periods of time in space. The testing of the Salyut 7/Soyuz T/Kosmos complex was the precursor to the third-generation space station "Mir." The Soviets had enhanced their capability and skill for EVA, and refined construction, inflight repair, and refueling techniques in space. These skills will prove invaluable for future, more complex space operations.

CURRENT ACTIVITIES IN SOVIET MANNED SPACE FLIGHT

The Generation Space Station: Mir

Currently, the Soviet Union is constructing a multimodular space complex with research directed toward hardware and life support systems that will permit man to exist safely in space for months and, perhaps, even years. This third generation space station, the Mir ("Peace"), represents the next step in a progressive space station program initiated in 1971. With the Mir, the Soviet Union has launched a total of eight space stations, each representing a substantial improvement over its predecessors.

The core of the Mir was launched February 20, 1986, the first stage of a new modular space station complex. The core vehicle has six docking ports for manned or unmanned capsules traveling to and from Earth. Four Kosmos-type dedicated laboratory modules will be docked to the core, enabling inflight studies in astrophysics, technological production, biological research, and medicine. Two axial ports can accommodate Soyuz vehicles or Progress resupply ships. The new space station also features improved crew facilities: private quarters, better windows, improved communications, an upgraded life support system, improved galley and food heating system with high quality dehydrated foods, and increased station automation (Ref. 9).

Unlike Salyut, the core module will be used mainly as a crew habitat, as most of the work stations will be located in the dedicated Kosmos laboratory modules. The crew area is thus much more spacious than before. The main computer complex, also located in the core, is more sophisticated and capable of running the space station automatically and autonomously.

On March 13, 1986, Cosmonauts Kizim and Solovyev, who set an endurance record of 237 days in space in 1984 on Salyut 7, were launched in their Soyuz T-15 vehicle to become Mir's first occupants. Their first task onboard Mir was initial activation and checkout of the station systems.

On May 6, the cosmonauts returned to the Salyut to perform several tasks left uncompleted when the last crew left quickly in November, 1985. This was the first flight between space stations. The Soyuz T-15 docked with Salyut 7 after flying from the Mir station. The transfer was regarded as a major accomplishment, opening new possibilities for servicing space stations in the future (Ref. 10).

An improved version of the Soyuz T spacecraft was launched May 21 and docked two days later with the Mir. The new vehicle, which flew without a crew, is designated Soyuz TM (M = modified). It later returned to Earth for reliability tests.

Salyut 7 cosmonauts performed an EVA on May 28 to construct a pylon in space. This 3-hour, 50-minute space walk brought the cumulative EVA time to over 24 hours for each individual. The cosmonauts spent 125 days in orbit before returning to Earth.

Soyuz TM-2 was launched February 6, 1987, carrying Cosmonauts Romanenko and Laveikin -- the second set of occupants of the Mir. The first dedicated module, an astrophysics module designated "Quantum," was launched March 31. After two failed docking attempts, the module finally docked with the core unit April 12, after the cosmonauts removed a foreign object during a 3-hour 40-minute EVA. This "rescue" of the module once again illustrates the utility and value of man in space.

With the new astrophysics module, the Soviets have begun specialized scientific work. In coming years, the assembled space station will resemble a large, rotating cross, with a mass of over 100 tons. In addition, work continues on extending crew time in space. With a one-year bed rest study already completed (including an evaluation of exercise, pharmaceutical, and dietary countermeasures) crewmembers on board the Mir may attempt stays of up to a year or more in preparation for bolder missions in the future (Ref. 11).

SOVIET SPACE MEDICINE TODAY

Biomedical Activities

As in the U.S., problem and research areas have been defined in the Soviet program on the basis of experience gained from 25 years of space flight. These include:

o   Microgravity effects on the body (space motion sickness, cardiovascular and muscle deconditioning, hematological changes, bone mineral loss) and necessary countermeasure development

o   Psychological factors (interior colors, crew comfort, work/rest cycle, isolation, entertainment, human factors, and tools)

o   Sociological challenges

o   Cosmic radiation

o   Space habitat/toxicology.

The biomedical preparation of cosmonauts has evolved considerably since the beginning of Soviet manned space flight, moving from a process that increased human tolerance of space flight factors to a network of interrelated measures designed to prepare cosmonauts physically and psychologically for life in space. This evolution was necessitated by the increasing complexity of space missions, as the role of the cosmonaut progressed from that of relatively passive passenger to operator performing complex tasks (including EVA) during long-term space flight. The following measures are currently included in the biomedical preparatory process (Ref. 12):

o   Medical selection and annual evaluations

o   General training

o   Specific (physiological/psychological) training

o   Medical training of prime and visiting flight crews

o   Medical care during flight

o   Postflight rehabilitation and therapy.

Protective Countermeasures

Because many physiological changes in space can be medically significant on return to Earth, the goal of countermeasures is to prevent complete adaptation to microgravity. Attempts to reduce and control the effects of weightlessness on cardiovascular and muscular deconditioning and bone demineralization have involved inflight, reentry, and postflight measures. Interventions have included inflight exercise, lower body negative pressure, fluid and electrolyte supplements, and antigravity suits. Additionally, nutritional supplements and pharmaceuticals have been tried on an experimental basis. The Soviets feel that many of these countermeasures have appreciable benefits (Ref. 13). However, the full extent of their effectiveness is not known. A variety of exercises, conditioning equipment, and methods that have found places on board Soviet spacecraft are described briefly in Table 1.

Table 1
COUNTER MEASURES USED ON SOVIET SPACE STATIONS

Exercise: 2-4 hrs/day for 6 days/week, divided into two sessions. Bicycle ergometer and treadmill with equipment for pulling loads parallel and perpendicular to long axis of body.

Penguin Suit: Places axial compression on musculoskeletal system. Worn throughout waking hours (8 hours/day).

Chibis Suit: Lower body negative pressure vacuum suit used for short periods in flight for tests. Regularly used 2-4 weeks before to Earth (to stress cardiovascular system).

Salt and Water Loading: Swallowing 3 g sodium chloride in 400 ml. water three times on day of recovery (to increase blood volume and prevent orthostatic intolerance). Used with Chibis suit.

Nutrition: Daily vitamins, caloric content.

Drugs: For skeletal protection.

Exercise Programs. During the past 15 years, durations of Soviet space missions have increased from days to months. Perhaps the most significant finding of the Salyut program was that physiological deconditioning can be substantially reduced through a regimen of vigorous exercises requiring 2-4 hours per day. Cosmonauts on longer missions using a prescribed physical training regimen have returned to Earth in generally good physical condition, showing swifter readaptation to one gravity (Ref. 14). Thus, prolonged human presence in space has become an operational reality, although physiological problems have by no means been eliminated.

The Soviets have required cosmonauts to exercise 2-4 hours per day (divided into sessions) for 6 days per week on the more recent Salyut flights. Some of these exercises were performed with a bicycle ergometer rated for increasing physical loads (Ref. 8). The treadmill exercises consisted of pulling loads parallel and perpendicular to the longitudinal axis of the body. Cosmonauts were monitored telemetrically not only for the load utilized and distance covered on the treadmill, but also for vital signs during exercise. Although variations in the frequency and duration of the exercise regimen have been dictated by mission details and cosmonaut desires, strenuous physical exercise during space flight remains an important countermeasure in the Soviet program for reducing the difficulties of readaptation to Earth's gravity (Ref. 14, 8).

Penguin Suit. The Penguin suit is a suit with bands of rubber woven into the fabric which, in response to movement, produces tension on various muscle groups of the legs and torso (Ref. 4). Worn during waking hours, the Penguin suit places an axial compression on the musculoskeletal system, requiring the cosmonaut to work against the suit to maintain an upright posture.

Chibis Suit/Salt Water Loading. Prior to the termination of long-duration space flight cosmonauts begin to use a lower body negative pressure suit called the Chibis vacuum suit (Ref. 15, 4). The negative pressure applied to the lower half of the body creates a downward redistribution of body fluids. The intent is to reestablish vascular tone for subsequent postflight orthostatic stability. Throughout the 2-4 week period before return to Earth, negative pressure is applied on a regular basis (every few days for a predetermined length of time). During the final two days of flight, negative pressure exposure is extended. During this phase, cosmonauts also drink about 400 ml. of water with 3 gm of sodium chloride (three times on day of recovery) before donning antigravity suits. The antigravity suit is worn prior to descent in order to create additional pressure to the lower extremities, preventing the pooling of blood in that area immediately after landing, and providing more rapid orthostatic compensation. The Chibis suit has also been used for brief periods inflight for test purposes.

Nutrition. Soviet observations indicate that both a regular meal schedule and acceptable foods are very important for the maintenance of optimum work capacity. Intervals of 15 to 20 minutes are allowed between exercise and intake of food, and 1 to 1.5 hours between food intake and initiation of exercise (Ref. 1). Caloric consumption on board the Salyut station average 3200 kcal. Soviet crews on long-term Salyut missions have generally maintained stable body weight. During the fourth Salyut 6 mission (185 days) cosmonauts actually gained weight, which they attributed to preventive measures including prescribed exercise, intake of vitamins twice daily, calcium supplements, body rehydration prior to landing, and appetite stimulators such as sharp seasonings (Ref. 5).

Drugs. Pharmacologic protection has been under extensive investigation for many years. In the area of radiation protection, protective compounds have been tested on experimental animals and humans. None are without side effects and their use is still experimental (Ref. 7). Diphosphonates offer some protection against bone demineralization, and show some promise. Among the approaches considered to prevent or reduce space motion sickness are prophylactic and/or therapeutic medications consisting primarily of central anticholinergic-acting drugs that augment central sympathetic activity (Ref. 1).

Postflight Recovery Activities

After long-duration flight, the first day postflight is characterized by considerable orthostatic intolerance and reliance on antigravity suit protection. The second day, however, crewmembers returning from missions as long as 237 days have walked with assistance, and by the fourth day, some light work was possible. The Soviets have employed physical exercise, physiotherapy, and psychotherapy to help cosmonauts readjust to Earth gravity (Ref. 14, 7). Supervised rehabilitation includes measures to restore the cardiovascular and musculoskeletal systems through walking, swimming, massage, special diets, and outdoor activity (Ref. 14). Postflight medical analyses continue for up to one month and include blood and urine analyses, bone/muscle tomography, and vestibular tests (chairs and parallel swings).

CONCLUSION

Throughout the history of the Soviet space program, space medicine has played a vital role in shaping the progress of Soviet manned space flight. Building on past experience and knowledge, the Soviet space medicine effort has become broad, comprehensive, and forward-looking.

Data from their manned missions clearly indicate that the Soviets have a keen appreciation of the biomedical problems encountered in space. The Soviet space station program has provided sophisticated facilities to investigate the long-term influence of microgravity on human physiology. Many of the observed biomedical deviations, such as bone demineralization, cardiovascular deconditioning, muscle atrophy, motion sickness, and terrestrial readaptation can only be quantified and investigated under actual space flight conditions.

In view of the physiological problems that may be encountered during extended space missions, it is critical that certain countermeasures be developed if manned space missions beyond one year are to become a reality. The Soviets are actively pursuing studies to this end. A one-year bed rest study, incorporating countermeasures, has already been completed (Ref. 16). Results of such studies, as well as the continued completion of long-duration missions, may provide the necessary knowledge to proceed with greater confidence toward further extending human stay-time and productivity in space.

REFERENCES

1. Nicogossian, A., and Parker, J.F., Jr. *Space Physiology and Medicine,* NASA SP-447, National Aeronautics and Space Administration, Washington, D.C., 1982, pp. 17-24.

2. Office of Technology Assessment: "Salyut: Soviet Steps Toward Permanent Human Presence in Space," OTA-TM-ST1-14, GPO no. 052-003-00937-4, Washington, D.C., December 1983.

3. Malyshev, Yu. "Evolution of the Soyuz Spacecraft," JPRS, USSR Report: Space, 2 March 1981, pp. 8-13.

4. Mumanskiy, S.P. "Cosmonaut Equipment" (translation of "Snaryazheniye Kosmonavta," Machinostroyeniye, Moscow, pp. 1-126, 1982), NASA TM-77192, Washington, D.C., February 1983.

5. U.S. Congress. Senate. Committee on Commerce, Science, and Transportation. Soviet Space Programs: 1976-1980, Part 2 (Suppl. 1983), U.S. Government Printing Office, Washington, D.C., October 1984.

6. Gurovsky, N.N., Kosmolinskiy, F.P., and Mel'nikov, L.N. Designing the Living and Working Conditions of Cosmonauts (translation of "Proyektirovaniye Usloviy Zhizni i Raboty Kosmonavtov," Machinostroyeniye, Moscow, pp. 1-168), NASA TM-76497, Washington, D.C., May 1981.

7. Bluth, B.J. and Helppie, M. "Soviet Space Stations as Analogs," 2nd edition, NAGW 69, NASA Headquarters, Washington, D.C., August 1986.

8. Hooke, L., Radtke, M., Garshnek, V., Teeter, R., and Rowe, J. A Physician on the Flight Crew (translation from *Zemlya I Vselennaya,* 5: 49-57, 1985). USSR Space Life Sciences Digest, NASA CR-3922 (05), 5: 1-8, 1986.

9. "Press Conference with Soyuz T-15/Mir/Salyut 7 Cosmonauts," *Soviet Aerospace,* August 1986.

10. "Cosmonauts Complete Transfer Between Mir and Salyut 7," *Aviation Week and Space Technology,* May 1986, p. 28.

11. Lomanov, G., "Whither Fly the Terrestrial Starships?" Sostialisticheskaya Industriya (in Russian), August 1986, p. 4.

12. Skibis, I.A., Tarasova, I.K., and Kalinichenko, V.V. "Biomedical Preparation of Cosmonauts," USSR Space Life Sciences Digest, L. Hooke et al. (eds.), NASA CR-3922(10), 9: 89, 1987.

13. Gazenko, O.G., Genin, A.M., and Yegorov, A.D. "Summary of Medical Investigations in the USSR Manned Space Missions," *ACTA Astronautica,* 8, 1981, pp. 907-917.

14. Krupina, T.N., Beregovkin, A.V., Bogolyubov, V.M., Fedorov, B.M., Yegorov, A.D., Tizul, A. Ya., Bogomolov, V.V., Kalinichenko, V.V., Ragulin, A.P. and Stepin, V.A. "Combined Rehabilitation and Therapeutic Measures in Space Medicine," *Sovietskaya Meditsina* (Moscow) 12: 3-8, December 1981.

15. Gazenko, O.G., and Yegorov, A.D. "The 175-Day Space Flight," *Moscow Vestrik Akademii Nauk SSSR,* 9:49-59, 1980.

16. *Tass* in English, 1300 gmt, "Research into Prolonged Hypokinesia," Nedelya, 10 April 1987.

RADIATION HAZARDS IN LOW EARTH ORBIT, POLAR ORBIT, GEOSYNCHRONOUS ORBIT, AND DEEP SPACE

Percival D. McCormack[*]

The predicted doses to the blood forming organs and skin of spacecraft crews in low inclination low Earth orbit, at high inclination and polar orbits, in geosynchronous orbit, and in free space are reviewed. Doses from trapped solar radiation and galactic cosmic radiation are covered, and also those to be expected from anomalous, large solar particle events. They are compared with the maximum annual and career doses laid down by the National Council on Radiation Protection (based on an excess lifetime risk of cancer of 3×10^{-2}). The effect of spacecraft and space suit shielding is also considered, along with the relative effectiveness of various shielding materials.

Shuttle flights have allowed extensive comparison of predicted doses with those measured experimentally. This has revealed some defects in the radiation and magnetic field models used and has led to extensive reexamination of these models.

INTRODUCTION

A central issue in manned space flight is the danger to the safety and health of humans caused by the ionizing radiation environment during long-term missions in space. The nature of the hazard varies with location and the major categories are:

a.   Low Earth orbit (altitude under 1,000 km and inclination below 40°)

b.   Geosynchronous orbit (altitude in vicinity of 37,000 km)

c.   Polar orbit (altitude under 1,000 km and 90° inclination)

d.   Deep space (including the Mars and lunar surfaces and Earth-Mars voyage).

In LEO, the major radiation hazard comes from the trapped protons in the South Atlantic Anomaly. These are largely high-energy protons with energies over 30 NeV and with quality factor of 1.2 (the proton differential spectrum is shown in Figure 1). There is a small constant background of galactic cosmic radiation (GCR), consisting of 81% protons, 14% alpha particles, and 1% heavy ions, with energies up to 10^{16} NeV (nuclear). Quality factors for this component can increase to over 20. Fluences vary by a factor of about 2.5 between Solar Min. and Solar Max. Low-altitude, low-inclination orbits are sheltered from solar particle events (solar flare activity).

---

[*]   Dr. McCormack is Manager, Operational Medicine, Life Sciences Division, NASA Headquarters, 600 Independence Ave., S.W., Washington, D.C. 20546.

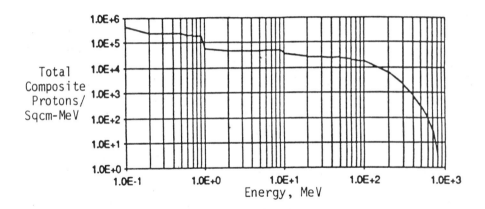

Figure 1 Proton Differential Spectrum

In GEO, the main radiation hazard is from trapped electrons which in traversing significant shield material will transform to bremsstrahlung. The quality factor for electrons and bremsstrahlung is about 1. There is also the GCR contribution referred to above. In polar orbit, spacecraft will encounter the South Atlantic Anomaly -- mainly protons -- the "horn" region of the outer electron belt, auroral electrons, and GCR. Finally, in deep space the radiation environment is primarily the GCR.

In the case of high-inclination LEO, polar orbit, GEO, and deep space, the greatest acute threat to humans is the solar particle event (SPE) -- that is, that solar flare actively associated with the emission of high-energy ionizing particles. SPEs are transient in nature, occur randomly (and almost exclusively during the Solar Max. period) and consist of protons and alpha particles with energies in the range from a few keV to several hundred MeV. The anomalously large event (AL) can deliver over 600 rem to the blood-forming organs (BFO) which would be acutely lethal. Such events occur at a frequency of 1 to 2 every 4 years. The AL event of August 1972 would have delivered 960 rem with no shielding. This threat and possible countermeasures will be considered in some detail later in this paper. The chronic exposure (relatively low level) scenarios will also be dealt with, but under the location headings "LEO", "GEO", "Polar Orbit," and "Deep Space" -- as described above.

BIOLOGICAL EFFECTS OF IONIZING RADIATION

Only chronic (long-term, low-level) effects will be considered, as acute (short-term, high-level) effects are well documented in the literature.

The biological effect of ionizing radiation on the blood-forming organs (considered, on the average, to lie at 5 cm of tissue below the skin) depends both on the amount of energy deposited in the tissue and the relative biological effectiveness (RBE) of the radiation:

Dose equivalent (REM) = RBE x dose (rads).

The RBE of different particle species is highly variable. It depends on the <u>rate</u> at which a particle deposits energy in tissue (LET); the distribution of energy deposited in a cell; the rate at which the dose is received, and the type of biological damage considered. Neutrons and heavy ions (e.g., iron) have RBEs of 10 and more for many biological actions. Cosmic ray iron nuclei deposit energy in cells at 600 times the concentration that cosmic ray protons do. Moreover, iron nuclei have an RBE about 20 times greater than protons for inducing cancers. Therefore, a rare cosmic ray iron nucleus is 12,000 times as dangerous as a cosmic ray proton.

Much research into the biological effects of heavy ions is underway. RBEs for specific biological endpoints in humans is often unknown. There is no accepted methodology at present for computing the overall health risk of a specific dose of radiation. For practical purposes, an (energy-dependent) quality factor is assigned to each particle species. Minimum ionizing radiations such as gamma rays and bremsstrahlung are assigned a quality factor of 1. The quality factors for heavy ions vary from 1 to 20; for secondary protons, $Q = 1.2$; for neutrons and nuclear recoils, $Q = 20$.

The biological effects which are of primary concern are:

1. Life-shortening effects, such as <u>carcinogenesis, mutagenesis</u>

2. Cataractogenesis

3. Genetic effects due to exposure of <u>reproductive tissue</u> (embryonic, fetal).

The development of career limits, as published in NCRP, is based on a lifetime excess risk of cancer (leukemia, lymphoma) of 3×10^{-2}. Such a lifetime risk is comparable to the risks in occupations such as construction and agriculture, but is greater than for terrestrial radiation-exposed workers. A 3% lifetime excess risk of death from cancer seems reasonable.

The latest limits laid down by the NCRP differentiate on the basis of age and sex for the career dose to the BFOs -- see Table 1 adapted from Ref. 1. They also take account of the risk for lymphoma induction (and not just for leukemia, as heretofore).

Table 1
CAREER LIMIT (rem) [a],[b]

Lifetime Excess Risk of Fatal Cancer	Age at first exposure	25	35	45	55
3×10^{-2}	Male	150	250	325	400
	Female	100	175	250	300

[a] Divide by 100 for dose equivalents in Sv.
[b] Based on a 10y exposure duration.

TRAPPED RADIATION EXPOSURE -- LOW-ALTITUDE, LOW-INCLINATION ORBITS (SPACE STATION AND SHUTTLE)

Magnetic Field Changes

The Earth's magnetic field is decaying slowly and the expected change in field strength between 1964 and 1994 is expected to be about 2.5%. There is considerable discussion at present on how to accommodate the change and to predict the radiation environment at Space Station Initial Operating Configuration (IOC) in 1994. Basically the question is whether to use the magnetic field model updated to 1994 or to use the magnetic field model that was valid at the time the AP8 model was created. As will be seen later, the two techniques result in very different predicted doses. Does the adiabatic inwards movement of the radiation, due to the decrease in magnetic field strength, dominate the atmospheric effects (which are independent of the magnetic field model)?

Trapped Radiation Models

The radiation model was compiled from data obtained by detectors flown on satellites within a few years of 1964 for the AP8-Min. and of 1970 for AP8-Max. (Ref. 2). For electrons, the AE8 model is used (Ref. 3). Note: the AE5 and AE8 models are the same for low Earth orbit and at low inclinations.

It is normal to represent radiation models as fluxes of particles of different species and energies, and to express their position in the magnetosphere as a function of McIlwain's L parameter and the magnetic field strength B (Ref. 4). To tie the radiation model to physical positions above the Earth's surface, one needs a magnetic field model which allows connection of the physical positions in terms of geographic longitude, latitude, and altitude with the B and L parameters. Use of valid magnetic field models, such as IGRF 1975, Barraclough 1975 (Ref. 5), AWC 1975, etc., with AP8 and AE8 should yield particle fluxes as a function of epoch, height, and geographic coordinates.

The magnetic field models also include time derivatives of the field expansion parameters, which permits some extrapolation into the future. All the models predict a decrease in the strength of the Earth's dipole. If AP8 is combined with a magnetic field which has been projected into the future, the apparent atmospheric cut-off will be depressed in altitude, and as the flux extinction is almost exponentially dependent on the altitude, the apparent radiation flux as a fixed altitude in the atmospheric cut-off will increase dramatically.

But fluxes below about 1000 km are subject to attenuation by the atmosphere, and this atmospheric attenuation layer is independent of the magnetic field. As this effect is not included in AP8, a projection of this model into the future might be expected to produce excessively high dose predictions. That this is indeed the case will be seen later.

In the Shuttle flights it has been possible to compare dose predictions and dosimetry results, and the next section will deal with this.

The final model, used by all Centers, is the MDAC (McDonnell Douglas Aerospace Corporation) man model developed for NASA Johnson Space Center (JSC). It is called Computerized Anatomical Man (CAM) (Ref. 6). For an isotropic radiation environment, this model allows computation of skin, eye, blood-forming organs, and gonad dose.

Shuttle (STS) Dose Calculations and Measurements

The Shuttle crew compartment was modeled as a 35 ft x 15 ft cylinder, or equivalent sphere with an absorption thickness of 2.0 g/cm^2 aluminum equivalent. The dose to a man target (in millirem per day) was computed for a range of altitudes from 150 to 325 nautical miles. Calculations were carried out at Goddard Space Flight Center (E. Stassinopoulos) with projection of the magnetic field model into the future, and by Johnson Space Center (A. Hardy) with no such projection. The JSC results are plotted in Figure 4 (skin dose only reported) along with observations from Shuttle flights. Best agreement with the Shuttle observations is obtained when no projection of the magnetic field into the future is carried out and for a Solar Max. situation -- although for the period in which these flights took place, Solar Min. is the appropriate situation. The GSFC results for the cylindrical model and Solar Min. are:

o   Approximately 6 times the JSC results for Solar Min., and

o   Approximately 10 times the JSC results for Solar Max. and the Shuttle dosimeter measurements.

Figure 2 shows dosimeter (TLD) locations in the aft flight deck of the Shuttle, and Figure 3 shows the location of the depth of dose rate meter and locations of dosimeters carried by the crewmen. Figure 4 shows the JSC computations of log dose (mrad/day) versus altitude for Solar Min. and Solar Max., compared with the Shuttle dosimeter measurements at location number 4. The agreement with the Solar Max. results is clearly the best.

Note: The constant contributions from the GCR has been included in both cases. Only the solar proton contribution is included, as the solar electron contribution is relatively small.

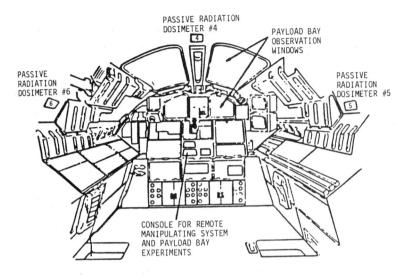

Figure 2   Dosimeter Locations - Aft Flight Deck

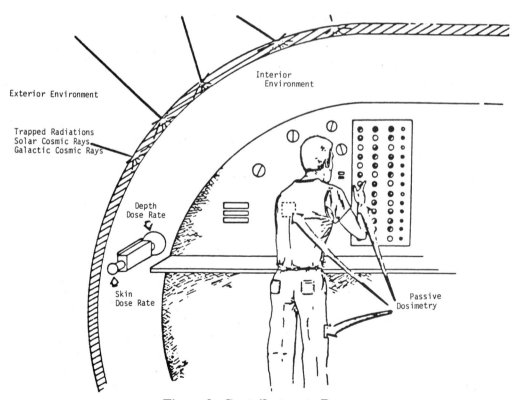

Figure 3   Contributors to Dose

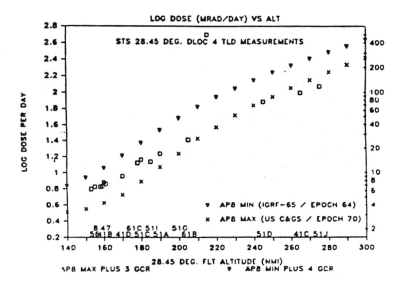

Figure 4 STS DLOC 4 Measurement Comparison

Assessment of Orbital Flux Integration Procedures

In order to resolve the issue of the large differences in calculated radiation dose levels between results based on updating the magnetic field to the IOC time frame and those based on no update, a panel of the foremost scientists in the field was convened at NASA Headquarters on February 25, 1986.

The Goddard Space Flight Center representative (E.G. Stassinopoulos) presented an outline of the procedures used at the Center in orbital radiation studies. These include:

o   Generation of a nominal flight path ephemeris

o   Selection of the simulated orbit time and integration of step size to provide sufficient point density along the orbit; and

o   Conversion of the trajectory from geodetic polar to magnetic B-L coordinates with McIlwain's INVAR program (Ref. 7) and the subroutine ALLMAG (Ref. 8) which utilizes either the Barraclough 1975 or the IGRF-80 field model.

The field computations are normally performed with expansion coefficients extrapolated to the indicated mission epoch using the secular variation terms of the models. The instantaneous positional charged particle fluxes are then obtained from current standard NASA models, using the version appropriate to the phase of the solar cycle -- Max. or Min. It must be noted that these are static environmental models. Orbital flux integrations are being simultaneously performed. Stassinopoulos pointed out that the change with time in the field strength B at a given physical position in the near-Earth domain places that position into a region of B-L

65

space that is associated with higher flux values in the static environment models. He would prefer a model adjustment (as proposed by Vette -- see later) rather than to arbitrarily omit updating the magnetic field.

The JSC representatives (A. Konradi, S. Nachtwey, and A. Hardy) then outlined their procedures. These are outlined in the block diagram shown in Figure 5. In Figure 6 proton flux is plotted versus altitude for periods starting with the epoch of the model and extrapolating forward as far as 2025. The increase in dose at a given altitude as the time period increases is clearly seen. It is also clear that projection to periods around 1995 and later produces the absurd result of positive fluxes at negative altitudes.

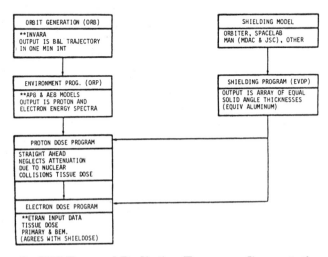

Figure 5   JSC Trapped Radiation Exposure Computations

The consensus reached by the experts is summarized as follows:

o   Adiabatic theory, which is the basis for contemporary radiation dose calculations, predicts that at altitudes below about 1,000 km there should be a change in the radiation environment from Solar Min. to Solar to Min. and (Max. to Max.). Experiment observations show that is not the case.

o   The source of the above anomaly is considered to lie in the considerable attenuation of radiation fluxes by the residual atmosphere at altitudes below 1,000 km or so. This atmospheric attenuation layer is independent of the magnetic field, but varies with the solar activity. As the constancy of this layer is not included in AP8 (or AE8), a secular projection of this model into the future will result in overestimation of the radiation dose.

o   The good agreement between Shuttle dosimetry and the JSC calculations, as outlined earlier, suggests that, fortuitously, magnetic field change effects and atmospheric change effects virtually cancel one another at these altitudes.

o   The unanimous recommendation of the panel was that, on an interim basis, dose calculations for the Space Station in the 1990 to 2000 period be based on:

-   Use of the AP8 Max. and Min. models with one of the reputable magnetic field models for the epoch 1970 and 1964, respectively.

-   No projection of the magnetic field into the future.

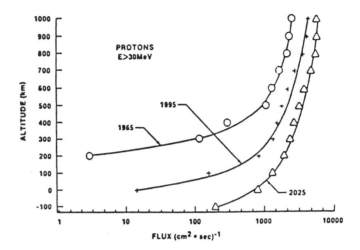

Figure 6 AWC 1975 S.A.A.

Model Adjustment Alternative

As Stassinopoulos has suggested, and the scientific community at large would prefer, a suitable model adjustment is required to account for the population depletions, rather than the arbitrary step detailed above. Such an adjustment has been made by Vette and Sawyer (Ref. 9) and will now be briefly described.

The geomagnetic field has been changing with time for over 86 years. The rate during the last 40 years has been between 16 and 30 nT (nano-Tesla). Most of this is due to dipole moment and the rest to higher moments. The question then arises as to the best way to calculate the trapped radiation fluxes using the AP8 and AE8 models. Nearly all the data used in making these models was organized into the B-L coordinate system using the magnetic field model of Jensen and Cain (Ref. 10) with an epoch of 1960. The value of the dipole strength for this year was .311653 gauss. Note: In geomagnetism the moment is divided by the Earth's radius cubed to produce the same units as magnetic field strength-gauss. In the computation of the parameter L, one should use the correct magnetic dipole. Everyone uses some version of McIlwain's INVAR routine. In the subroutine CARMEL there are two places where the constant .311653 appears. These should be replaced by the dipole moment of the model that is being used to compute B and L. Using Hilton's formulation for the F functions used to compute L from B and I (Ref. 11), there are four places to insert the proper dipole moment.

From the formulation of L it will be seen that L is nearly independent of M (dipole moment). The quantity B/B_0 is also nearly independent of M -- it is only a function of magnetic latitude in the dipole case. The L, B/B_0 pair as thus described should be virtually independent of time (B_0 is the equatorial B value). These will yield J $(L,E.B/B_o)$ values that are also nearly constant with time (E is the energy and J is the omnidirectional flux at energies greater than E). Preliminary results obtained by Sawyer and Vette indicate that proton fluxes decrease by about 10% at Space Station altitudes for the period of 1964 to 1986. Generally, the various Centers have been performing calculations for new epochs but retaining M = .311653. As this results in a lower B value and a slightly higher L, the J values increase with time at Space Station altitudes -- and this is an artifact of the calculation.

There is little data available on the change in the Van Allen belt in the last 15 years -- this situation will change if the CRESS satellite is successful (late 1980s), and then a new meaningful trapped radiation model can be created. Sawyer and Vette have agreed to change the programs that they distribute to the scientific community, to enable the change recommended above to be carried out. This involves changing the subroutine TRARA1 to accept the triple (L,E,B,B_o) rather than (L,E,B) as input to the calculation of J from the models. Program MODEL will be modified to pass B/B_o to TRARA1. Program ORB will be modified to output B/B_o, as well as B, and to calculate L directly, using INVAR with a magnetic dipole moment fed into CARMEL that is consistent with the epoch of the magnetic field model. In this way it is hoped to avoid the pitfall of passing the dipole moment from one program to another and thus obtain reasonable flux values in calculating for epochs later than 1960. Ultimately, the accuracy of these flux values must await confirmation by new models based on satellite data.

Dose Predictions for Space Station

The common module in the Space Station will be cylindrical in shape-- 43.7 feet long and 14.8 feet in diameter -- see Figure 7. The wall is complex, consisting of the inner pressure shell, outer bumper layer, plus spacers. For the purpose of initial dose calculation a single pressure layer of aluminum, .125 inches thick, was assumed (.3175 cm or .86 gm/cm^2). The calculations were done for protons only, as the electron dose is negligible. Doses are given in millirem -- a quality factor of 1.2 was used. The models used were AP8-MIN, IGRF 1965 for epoch 1964, with a man target and AP8-MAX, Hurwitz (USC and GS) for epoch 1970 with a man target. The dose/day to the skin and blood-forming organs in Space Station crewmembers are shown in Figure 8. The rapid rise in dose at altitudes over 450 km is very obvious. The radiation exposure limits for astronauts, as presently formulated by the National Council for Radiation Protection (NCRP) are shown in Table 1. Table 2 shows nominal Space Station orbital parameters.

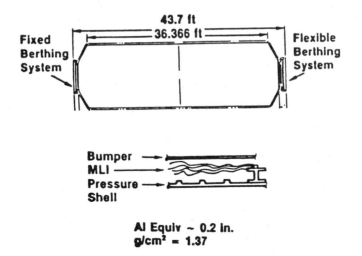

Figure 7   Common Module

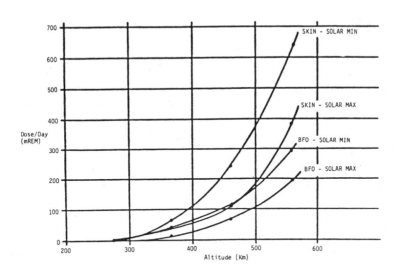

Figure 8   Predicted Dose Rate to Crewmembers is Space Station

69

Table 2
SPACE STATION ORBITAL PARAMETERS

Element	NOMINAL Altitude	Inclination (Degrees)	DESIGN ALTITUDE RANGE High	Low
Space Station	500 km (270 n. mi)	28.5	555 km (300 n. mi)	463 km (250 n. mi)
Co-Orbiting Platform(s)	500 km (270 n. mi)	28.5	1000 km (540 n. mi)	463 km (250 n. mi)
Polar Platform Platform(s)*	750 km (381 n. mi)	98.25	900 km (486 n. mi)	400 km (215 n. mi)

*Polar Servicing Altitude 276 km (149 n. mi)

For a 40-year-old male, for example, the career limit would be 275 rem to the BFO. Even with Solar Min. conditions, the astronaut could make a 3-month tour every 2 years over a 20-year career with no problem. For a 1-year stay during Solar Min. the dose would be 65 rem -- exceeding the annual limit. One way to overcome this would be to double the module wall thickness -- to about .25 inches aluminum. This would reduce the dose by a factor of 1.2 and the annual dose to just under the annual limit (see Figure 9).

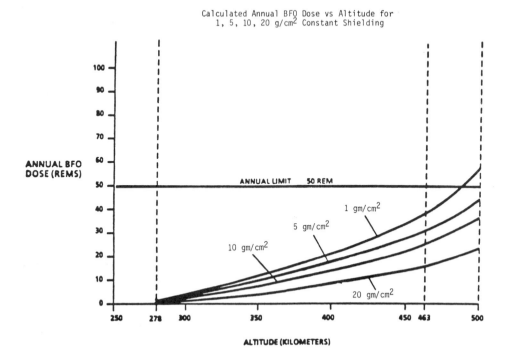

Figure 9   Annual BFO Dose for Space Station

Figure 9 also shows the yearly dose versus shield thickness. The module weight penalty would be about 3000 lbs. (see Figure 10). Increasing radiation protection by increasing wall thickness is an expensive countermeasure. Decrease in Space Station altitude during Solar Min. periods would be a much more economical measure (constant drag strategy).

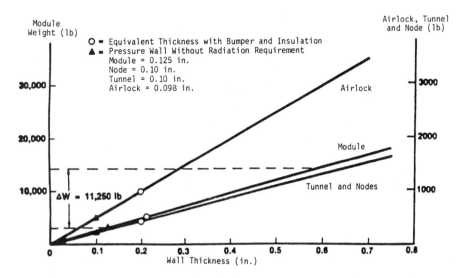

Figure 10 Module Shielding Penalty

The present dose calculation procedures for Space Station are the best available at this time. More realistic calculations will be done in the near future:

o   To account for the shielding provided by equipment and racks internal to the module;

o   To parametrically optimize the module wall assembly with respect to radiation shielding;

o   To account for the presence of windows; and,

o   To account for the nonisotropic nature of the radiation flux in low Earth orbit.

The EVA workload in Space Station will be heavy, and it will not be always possible to program EVAs to avoid intersection with the South Atlantic Anomaly. Figure 11 shows the shielding afforded by the present (Shuttle) space suit assembly. The shielding afforded is inadequate for Space Station EVA operations. In the more advanced space suits under development, shielding of over 1.5 g/cm^2 aluminum equivalent will be provided over the entire body and head of the crewman.

Further study of the biological effects of the neutron and high Z components of the cosmic radiation in LEO also must be carried out. Finally, as mentioned earlier, the data from the CRESS satellite and from Space Station itself will, in due course, enable more accurate radiation models to be formulated.

MATERIAL COVERING ARMS AND LEGS

	DENSITY (g/cm²)	THICKNESS (inches)
Thermal Management Garment (TMG)	.091	.053
Restraint-Dacron/Bladder Fabric	.035	.020
Liquid Cooling Ventilation Garment (LCVG)	.039	.0295
Total	.165	.1025

Approx. Alum equiv ~ .2 g/cm²

UPPER TORSO

TMG	.091	.053
Fiberglass Shell	.354	.075
LCVG	.039	.0275
Total	.484	.158

Approx. Alum. Equiv. ~ .5 g/cm²

EYE SHIELD

	DENSITY (g/cm²)	THICKNESS (inches)
Helmet Bubble	.182	.06
Protective Visor	.182	.06
Sun Visor	.190	.06
Center Eyeshades	.067	.07
Side Eyeshades	.238	.125
Total	.859	.375

Approx. Alum. Equiv. ~ 0.9 g/cm²

Figure 11   Space Suit Assembly (Shuttle) Shielding Values

RADIATION ENVIRONMENT AND EXPECTED ABSORBED DOSE IN GEO

A specific GEO orbit will be taken, to give a worst-case situation. Doses have been estimated for an orbital stay time of 15 days.

The main contributor to the absorbed dose is from <u>trapped electrons</u> at low shielding thickness (less than 2 g/cm^2 Al) and, at larger shielding thicknesses, from bremsstrahlung produced by the electrons.

The average daily dose will depend also on the parking orbit assumed. The most unfavorable parking longitude from a radiation exposure standpoint is 160 degrees W. There, the spacecraft would penetrate most deeply into the outer electron belt. The resultant dose to the BFO inside a spherical shell of thickness 2 g/cm^2 Al is 48 mrad/day or 0.7 rad for 15 days (Solar Min.). The average quality factor (Q) for electrons and bremsstrahlung is 1 and so the dose equivalent is 0.7 rem. This only drops by a factor of 2 if the shield thickness is increased to 5 g/cm^2 due to the persistence of the bremsstrahlung component. Note: Statistical variation occurs and depending on solar activity and magnetospheric conditions locally, radiation exposure higher than those presented above could occur.

GCR would add an increased dose of approximately 0.3 rad or an increased dose equivalent of 0.8 rem at Solar Min. These doses are subject to worked temporal variations.

The dose accumulated during traversal of the radiation belts from low- to high Earth orbit depends critically on the length of the time required to reach GEO altitude. Estimations of mission exposure for this scenario depend on trajectory chosen, means of propulsion, etc. A high-thrust rapid traversal trajectory (lasting 5.5 hours) might add, as a worst case, 2 rem to the BFO on each trip out and back through the trapped radiation belts.

Finally, occurrence of an anomalously large solar particle event could add, at 2 g/cm^2 Al shielding:

105 rem (85 rad) -- BFO

900 rem (650 rad) -- eyes

1100 rem (800 rad) -- skin

Increase in shielding to 10 g/cm^2 Al decreases:

BFO exposure to about 18 rem

Eye exposure to about 90 rem

Skin exposure to about 92 rem

The use of a Solar X-Ray Imager on a NOAA satellite would provide a 2-hour warning with 95% probability of SPE prediction. The deorbit option is not safe (within 2 hours the particle flux in GEO would rise to near peak value). There is no alternative but to provide a safe haven in GEO with a shield in the vicinity of 20 g/cm^2 Al.

POLAR ORBIT

It is estimated that the dose behind a 1 g/cm^2 Al shield at 450 km altitude to the BFO would be about 7 rem in 90 days (approximately 40% due to GCR). This falls to about 1.25 rem behind 2 g/cm^2 Al. Table 3 compares 90-day doses in LEO for low-inclination, medium-inclination, and polar orbits for 1 g/cm^2 Al shield. In polar orbits, spacecraft are also exposed to SPEs and the doses listed above for an AL event in GEO would apply to polar orbits also.

Table 3
DOSE ESTIMATES FOR SPACE MISSIONS IN LOW EARTH ORBIT (1.0 gm/cm^2 Al Shielding)

Mission	Radiation Source	Duration (Days)	Dose (Rem) Bone Marrow	Skin
LEO Space Station 450 km 28-1/2° Orbit	South Atlantic Anomaly Galactic Cosmic Rays	90	9	16
LEO Medium Inclination 450 km 57° Orbit	Galactic Cosmic Rays South Atlantic Anomaly	90	7	14
LEO Polar Orbit 450 km 90° Orbit	Galactic Cosmic Rays South Atlantic Anomaly	90	7	12

73

DEEP SPACE -- MARTIAN, LUNAR MISSIONS

Apart from SPEs, the major radiation to which astronauts will be subject on Martian or lunar missions is GCR. GCR energies can be very high, ranging to 10^{14} NeV (compared to 30 NeV for Solar particles). Such particles are very penetrating and can traverse over 10 meters of lunar soil (compared to 1 cm for solar particles). At a depth of 2.5 g/cm^2, the predicted dose during Solar Min. is about 47 rem per year. In a 3-year round trip to Mars, the expected dose behind 2-1/2 g/cm^2 would be about 140 rem to the BFO. This is substantial, but still below the lifetime limit set by the NCRP. It is also higher than it should be, as the dose received from GCR on the Martian surface would be halved by the shielding effect of the planet's mass. Of great concern, however, is exposure to the heavy ion component of GCR, which dominates the radiation dose equivalent for cancer induction.

The other important source of energetic particles outside the Earth's magnetosphere is solar flares. Flares deliver very high doses over short periods (a few hours or days). Without shielding, exposure to anomalously large events would be deadly to astronauts. But solar particle energies (as pointed out above) are much less than that of GCR, and are stopped by less shielding material. The characteristics of solar flares and the particles emitted will be considered in the next section.

SOLAR FLARES AND SOLAR PARTICLE EVENTS

Not all solar flare activity on the Sun results in particle emission, and even with particle emission these may not always be directed at the Earth. Those flares which satisfy both these criteria are termed Solar Particle Events (SPEs). SPEs occur at a rate of about 100 per 11-year solar cycle and predominantly during Solar Max. Unless the flux is over 10 protons/cm^2 -- sec -- steradian (or roughly 1 rad/hour) in the Earth's vicinity, the event is not regarded as AL. Most SPEs are below the alarm threshold. There are about 2-3 AL events in 4 to 6 years during Solar Max.

Prior to particle emission (impulsive phase) from the Sun (from 2 to 20 minutes) there is X-radiation emission (a precursor). SPEs are associated with hard X-ray emission. Visible emission occurs at roughly the same time as X-radiation, and lasts about 30 to 50 minutes. The electromagnetic outputs reach the Earth in about 8 minutes. The solar particles (mainly protons), depending on their energy, take from 30 to 100 minutes to reach the Earth. The time scale of events is summarized in Table 4. The solar proton flux remains elevated for 36 to 48 hours postflare.

Letaw (Ref. 12) reports the total dose in rem/hour for the August 1972 flare and a composite worst-case flare. It is seen that the August 1972 flare intensity is reduced to a tolerable level with 70 g/cm^2 shielding. Over the effective period 15.5 hours a dose of 2.2 rem is accumulated. The buildup of secondary particles from the worst-case flare, however, results in a total dose of 236 rem over the same period. Additional amounts of Al shielding will not reduce this very much. Heavy ions do not form the most important component dose to the BFO. The proton secondary component is approximately equal to its primary component between 20 g/cm^2 (7.5 cm Al) and 70 g/cm^2 (26 cm). The largest component is low energy (<20 Nev) neutrons. Table 5 shows the total dose (in rad) to the BFO at shielding of 2 g/cm^2 and .25 g/cm^2 (the average body shielding during EVA in a Shuttle space suit). Exposure to an AL event particle flux during EVA in a "soft" space suit would result in a lethal dose.

Table 4
TIME SCALE OF EVENTS

Event	XR + Visible Emission on Sun	XR + Visible Arrive Earth	Particles Emitted at Sun	Arrive at Earth
Time (minutes)	0	+8	+15	+45-->120

- Lead-time based on XR/visible observation 35 → 112 minutes
- Particle flux level ↑ over APP. 30 minutes to reach Max.
- Max evasion time available 65 → 142 minutes

Table 5
AVERAGE DAILY DOSE

o   160 nautical mile altitude Shuttle shielding ~ 2 g/cm^2

Inclination	Daily (M.Rad)	30 Days
28° --> 38°	5.2 --> 6.5	~180
57°	10.3	~310

o   200 nautical mile altitude

Inclination	4 g/cm^2	30-Day (Rad.) 2 g/cm2	.25 g/cm^2*
28,5°	1.8	2.4	30
90° (Polar)	1.8	6.0	

*EVA soft space suit shielding

STS Solar Flare Alarm System

The present alarm system consists of:

a. Ground-based optical and radio-telescopes

   -   USAF and NASA

b. Whole Sun X-ray detector on a NOAA GOES satellite

c. Space Environment Services Center (SESC), Boulder, Colorado. This has a computer program which makes SPE predictions based on information relayed from (a.) and (b.).

This system provides a 20-minute warning to the Shuttle, and with a possible 2-hour buildup to peak particle flux, would just about allow:

a. Termination of an EVA

b. Orientation of Shuttle "belly-up"

c. Deorbit to commence (to emergency landing sites, if necessary).

The present system has several defects:

a. Global cloud cover would eliminate the observatory system.

b. Solar flare visible output from behind the Sun's horizon cannot be seen.

c. The SESC SPE prediction capability is not very reliable (many false positives).

Use of a Solar X-Ray Imager on a NOAA satellite is being considered at present, to improve the solar flare alarm system. However, 5% false positives in SPE prediction will still occur, and there is no increase in the advance time of warning (X-ray and visible emission occur almost simultaneously). NASA plans to support increased solar physics study with a view to producing a more effective warning system.

On an Earth-Mars or Earth-Moon mission there is no option to deorbit and the only countermeasure to lethal SPEs is to provide the crew with a safe haven with at least 50 g/cm^2 equivalent Al protection all around.

SHIELDING COUNTERMEASURES

It has been indicated above that shielding in a solar flare shelter must be over 70 g/cm^2 equivalent. With the lower energy particles in SPEs, this should be reasonably satisfactory. However, even in this case parametric optimization of composite shield materials should be undertaken. Materials with high hydrogen content (water, polythylene, etc.) provide more effective shielding than aluminum -- see Figure 12. Alternate layers of tantalum and aluminum are also more effective than the same thickness of aluminum above.

Further studies of the composite worst-case flare environment, its radiobiological effect and procedures (possibly pharmaceutical) for protecting against flare absorbed doses during solar flares, must be carried out to minimize this serious hazard to humans in space.

Galactic cosmic radiation (GCR) shielding on spacecraft designed to carry humans into deep space during Solar Min. must be provided with habitable spaces shielded with at least 20 g/cm^2 (7.5 cm) Al (or shielding of equivalent effect.) It is more important in this case both economically and from the health risk point of view, to parametrically optimize the spacecraft shielding as discussed above. Moreover, racks and equipment on board the spacecraft provide considerable shielding (over 16 g/cm^2 in places) and maximum use of this inbuilt protection must be utilized.

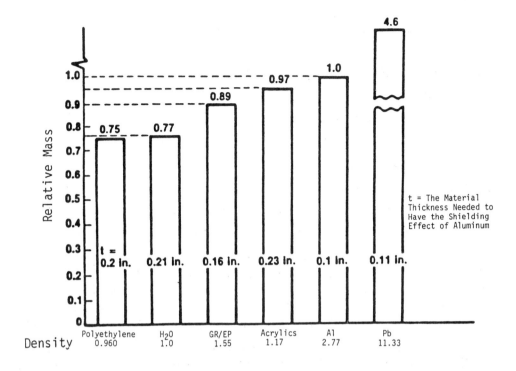

Figure 12 Material Shielding Values

The expected dose from GCR at Solar Min., with no shielding is 49 rem/year. This is within NCRP limits (50 rem/year) but with the uncertainty in the estimates one is forced to add shielding. With 20 g/cm^2 (7.5 cm) Al the exposed dose falls to 31 rem/year. Adding an additional 30 g/cm^2 would only reduce this by 5 rem/year. Hence the necessity for shielding optimization.

During Solar Max. the GCR dose equivalent is below 20 rem/year for all shielding thicknesses. NCRP limits are easily met during Solar Max.

After several years of flight in deep space (outside the magnetosphere) career dose limits for younger astronauts (less than 200 rem) will be attained. A 3-year mission to Mars at Solar Min. will produce an absorbed dose of 100 rem with the shielding recommended here. Astronauts over 40, with no previous space flights, are at the least risk on a Mars mission. Crew selection based on established genetic susceptibility to radiation damage may also become an ameliorating factor.

Note: On the lunar surface with no shielding, the BFO dose is about 30 rem/year; on the Martian surface it is about 12 rem/year.

CONCLUDING REMARKS

It is obvious that even on 3-year Mars voyages, the radiation dose to the crew can be kept below the lifetime doses as specified by the NCRP. Shuttle deorbit, improved flare warning system, composite shielding, and flare shelters can make known radiation risks acceptable for:

    a.   Year-long sojourns on Space Stations.

    b.   GEO and polar missions

    c.   Martian and lunar sojourns.

However, of great concern is the fact that neutrons and heavy ions have RBEs of over 10 for many biological end-effects. Carcinogenesis, mutagenesis, and cataractogenesis (and other analogous neural damage) due to these particles must be studied extensively in the years to come. An enhanced Radiobiology and Radiological Research Program has recently been formulated at NASA headquarters to meet the objective of shedding more light on these unknowns.

REFERENCES

1. *NCRP Report.* "Guidance on Radiation Received in Space Activities," 1987.

2. Sawyer, D. and Vette, J. "AP8 Trapped Proton Environment for Solar Max. and Solar Min.," Goddard Space Flight Center, 1976.

3. Teague, M.J. and Vette, J. "AE5 -- A Model of the Trapped Electron Population for Solar Min." NASA Goddard Space Flight Center, April, 1974.

4. McIlwain, G. "Coordinates for Mapping the Distribution of Magnetically Trapped Particles." *G. Geophys. Res. 66,* 1961, pp.187-194.

5. Barraclough, D.R., et al. "A Model of the Geomagnetic Field at Epoch 1975." *Geophys. R. Roy. Ast. Soc. 43,* pp645-659.

6. Billings, M.P. and Yucker, W.R. "The Computerized Anatomical Man" *(NASA CR 13403),* 1972.

7. Hassett, A. and McIlwain, C.G. "Computer Programs for the Computation of B&L." *Data Users Note NSSOC 67-27,* National Space Science Data Center, Greenbelt, Maryland, 1966.

8. Stassinopoulos, E.G., and Mead, G.D. "ALLMAG, GDALMG, LINTRA: Computer Programs for Geomagnetic Field and Field-line Calculation." *NSSDC 72-12,* National Space Science Data Center, Greenbelt, Maryland, 1972.

9. Sawyer, D. and Vette, J. (Private communication.) NASA Goddard Space Flight Center, 1986.

10 Cain, G.C. et al. "A Proposed Model for the International Geomagnetic Reference Field." *G. Geomag, Geoelec. 19,* 1967, pp335-355.

11. Hilton, H.J. *Geophysics Research, Vol. 76,* pp6652-6653, 1971.

12. Letaw, G. and Clearwater, S. "Radiation Shielding Requirements on Long Duration Missions." *Report SCC 86-02.* Severn Communications Corporation, 1986.

ASSESSMENT OF THE EFFICACY OF MEDICAL COUNTERMEASURES IN SPACE FLIGHT[*]

A.E. Nicogossian[†], F. Sulzman[†], M. Radtke[‡], and M. Bungo[**]

Changes in body fluids, electrolytes, and muscle mass are manifestations of adaptation to space flight and readaptation to the 1-g environment. The purposes of this paper are to review the current knowledge of biomedical responses to short- and long-duration space missions and to assess the efficacy of countermeasures to 1-g conditioning. Exercise protocols, fluid hydration, dietary and potential pharmacologic measures are evaluated, and directions for future research activities are recommended.

INTRODUCTION

With the emergence of the International Space Station Program, there has been renewed interest in the need for specific countermeasures to facilitate readaptation to 1-g. As the planning for the design of the Space Station and missions beyond the Earth's orbit proceeds, important issues such as environmental health, radiation protection, amount of physical conditioning, and selection and training of crews have resurfaced as focal points of discussion. These issues can profoundly affect the design of future space systems and set the pace for additional ground and flight experiments to be conducted well into the early era of Space Station operations. In this context, information obtained from short-duration Space Transportation System (STS) missions has proven to be of value in reassessing the knowledge gained from prior Skylab missions and in the formulation of some operation research strategies.

STS REVIEWED

All data were reviewed from the first 24 STS missions which had relevance to the assessment of the mechanisms involved in adaptation to space flight.

---

[*] Paper IAF/IAA 86-394 presented at the 37th Congress of the International Astronautical Federation, Innsbruck, Austria, 4-11 October 1986. The paper is reprinted with permission of Pergamon Press plc., from Acta Astronautica, Vol. 17, No. 2, pp 195-198, February, 1988.

[†] NASA Headquarters, Life Sciences Division, 600 Independence Ave., S.W., Washington, D.C. 20546.

[‡] Management and Technical Services Co., Washington, D.C.

[**] NASA Space Biomedical Research Institute, NASA Lyndon B. Johnson Space Center, Houston, Texas 77058.

Significant alterations were found in the neurovestibular systems (Table 1). Human studies indicated a total reinterpretation of perceived self-motion and variations in the metabolism of drugs. Changes in the cardiovascular system included early fluid shifts [1] starting on the launch pad (because of the head-down position while in the vertical launch configuration), lack of change in the intraocular pressure inflight, translocation of up to 1.21. of fluids from each leg with subsequent loss of total body fluids by the second day inflight, increased calcium loss, no changes in the vitamin D metabolites, maintenance of cardiac output at the expense of increased heart rate, increase in peripheral vascular resistance, and partial effectiveness of orally ingested normal saline solution which is taken to prevent postflight orthostatic intolerance (Tables 2 and 3). In addition, studies performed on rodents have shown significant rearrangement in the distribution of the fast- versus slow-twitch muscle fiber populations postflight.

Table 1
SUMMARY OF STS MEDICAL INVESTIGATIONS: NEUROLOGIC

o   The time course of space motion sickness (SMS) symptoms has been characterized.

o   No preflight predictors of SMS have been identified.

o   No correlation was found for fluid shifts and SMS.

o   No alterations were observed in visual acuity or performance.

o   All otolith displacements (e.g. head tilt) are reinterpreted as linear motion.

o   Drug efficacy is altered in space flight.

Table 2
SUMMARY OF STS MEDICAL INVESTIGATIONS: FLUID AND ELECTROLYTE

o   Fluid shifts start on the launch pad.

o   Total body water decreased by the second flight day.

o   No changes in intraocular pressure.

o   Potassium excretion rate is unchanged inflight.

o   Increased inflight excretion of sodium.

o   Serum concentration of calcium was decreased inflight.

o   No change in vitamin D metabolite concentrations.

Table 3
SUMMARY OF STS MEDICAL INVESTIGATIONS: CARDIOVASCULAR

o   Initial increase in central venous pressure slowly decreases by flight-day 3.

o   Decreased left ventricular end-diastolic volume index (LVDVI) and stroke volume index; increased peripheral vascular resistance.

o   Larger preflight LVDVI values correlate with postflight cardiac index of deconditioning (CID).

o   Normal saline ingestion partially improves the CID.

SKYLAB REVIEWED

With this new information in hand, a critical review of specific data from the three Skylab missions was conducted [2]. Heart rate and blood pressure responses of Skylab crewmembers were evaluated during lower body negative pressure (LBNP) tests, exercise using a bicycle ergometer, and personal daily exercise regimens. Comparison of muscle strength loss in the lower extremities during each mission, including loss of calcaneal mass, and overall weight changes were examined for potential correlations of cause and effect. Unfortunately, because of the small sample size (nine crewmembers) only general trends of association could be established.

The effect of the total exercise effort on leg strength in the three Skylab missions is shown in Fig. 1. During the first manned Skylab mission only the bicycle ergometer was used. During the second mission isokinetic devises MKI and II were added, and during the last and longest mission the treadmill was included in the overall daily exercise protocol. There was no significant change observed in postflight leg muscle strength between the first and second missions, while significant improvements were noted in all crewmembers in the last mission, where the treadmill was used. In addition, although Skylab 3 and 4 crews started at approximately the same preflight levels of physical conditioning (as determined by oxygen consumption), a distinct improvement in $\dot{V}_{O2}$ was noted during the last mission (Figure 2) [3].

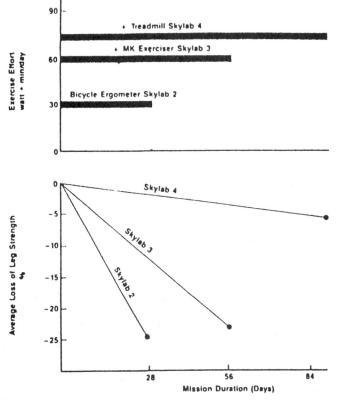

Fig. 1   Effect of Exercise on Leg Strength of Skylab Crews

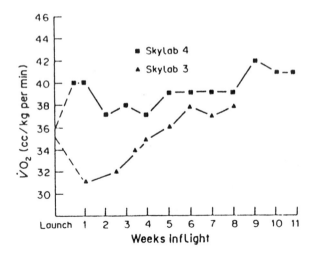

Fig. 2   Changes in Physical Conditioning During Skylab Missions

Earlier, it had been hypothesized that LBNP had a beneficial effect on the fitness level of astronauts, and suggestions were made to utilize this device for physical conditioning in future long-duration missions. A review of Skylab LBNP data, both at rest and at 50 torr negative pressure, showed a consistent increase in both resting and stressed heart rates throughout the flights. A tendency toward stabilization of the heart rate response was observed by the tenth day in Skylab, with a similar finding on STS (Figure 3). Further review of the LBNP data showed that the majority of crewmembers responded with a pronounced orthostatic response postflight (Figure 4). Only one crewmember on the Skylab 4 mission had a comparable response to his preflight tests (Figure 5). These data seem to indicate that although LBNP might have had some favorable effects on the crewmembers' tolerance to repeated passive cardiovascular stress as the flight progressed, only one crewmember demonstrated a beneficial postflight effect on his physical conditioning and orthostatic response.

It is well known that contractions of the antigravity muscles of the lower extremities help in the return of the blood to the right side of the heart. Atrophy of these muscles and changes in the ability to sustain isometric contractions can result in a decrement in postflight orthostatic tolerance, especially if combined with loss in circulating blood volume, which is the case in space flight. As shown on STS missions, there is a loss of total body fluids by the second day inflight, primarily due to reduced thirst, decrease in fluid intake due to motion sickness, and perhaps a late diuresis due to cepahalad fluid shifts.

Reduction of lower extremities muscle mass was coupled with fluid losses and changes in strength of the antigravity muscles, causing fluid pooling and a decrease in filling volume of the right side of the heart. The replenishment of intravascular fluid with isotonic solutions may not be a very effective countermeasure, since most of the fluid is transferred passively to the interstitial spaces.

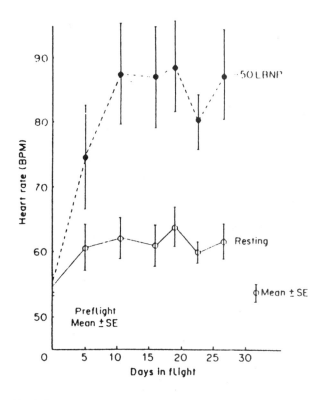

Fig. 3 Skylab 9-Man Average Heart Rate at Maximum LBNP

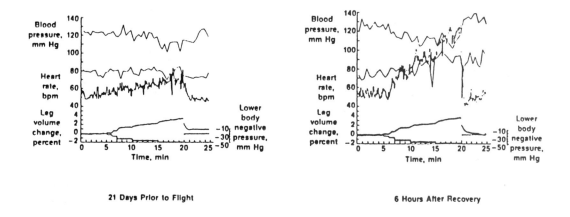

Fig. 4 Results of Lower Body Negative Pressure Tests
on Skylab 4 Scientist Pilot

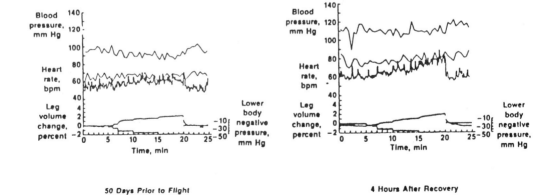

**Fig. 5   Results of Lower Body Negative Pressure Tests
on Skylab 4 Commander**

The individual responses of Skylab 4 crews to different types of exercise are shown in Table 4. Although the Commander performed the least work on the bicycle ergometer, he did not exhibit weight or os calcis mass losses postflight. Changes in his stressed heart level during maximum LBNP were also less pronounced than in the other two crewmembers. The main difference which could account for this response might be the walking and running on the treadmill and/or individual physical fitness which resulted in such a dramatic recovery response postflight.

Table 4
DAILY EXERCISE PROTOCOLS OF SKYLAB 4 CREW AND POSTFLIGHT RESPONSES

Exercise	Commander	Scientist pilot	Pilot
Leg ergometry (watt min)	5000	8337	6000
Treadmill:			
Walk (min)	10	0	0
Run (min)	1	0	0
Springs (repetitions)	300	1000	100
Toe rises (repetitions)	200	200	75
Postflight left os calcis	+0.7	−4.5	−7.9
% weight change	0	−3.7	−2.2
Inflight-preflight heart rate at −50 mm Hg	+12	+37	+27

CONCLUSIONS

Partial prevention of physiological adaptation to weightlessness seems a natural approach to preparing crewmembers to successfully cope with readaptation to 1-g conditions. It is now recognized that the cardiovascular system's adaptation to space flight proceeds in an appropriate fashion. Evidence of this normal adaptive process is provided by extravehicular activities which, while physically demanding, do not cause any cardiovascular decompensation. However, symptoms of orthostatic intolerance do appear upon return to Earth's gravitational field. The presence of orthostatic intolerance as a postflight syndrome depends largely on the loss of total body fluids and the functional state of antigravity muscles. However, certain alterations in motor reflexes may also pay a role. Motion sickness contributes to fluid losses, with secondary neurohumoral adjustments. Physical training sessions contribute fluid loss through perspiration.

Secondary effects of adaptive changes to space flight coupled with unabated urinary calcium excretion and increased urinary osmolality, if accompanied by an inappropriate diet, can have significant impacts on crew health, such as development of renal calculi. Sustained increases of calcium excretion in the urine, if unchecked, can result in the formation of renal stones. Table 5 summaries conditions which can be conducive to urinary tract stone formation. It should be noted that several of these conditions, such as negative water balance, sustained physical effort during exercise, and excessive excretion of some electrolytes and amino acids are present in space flight. Table 6 summaries urinary biochemical findings in Shuttle and Skylab missions [4]. Excretion of uric acid proteins, and electrolytes is largely dependent upon the composition of the diet consumed.

Table 5
INFLIGHT STONE RISK FACTORS

o   High level of exercise.

o   Dehydration.

o   High animal protein diets.

o   Increased saturation of stone-forming salts (calcium oxalate and calcium phosphate).

o   Reduced citrate excretion (stone inhibitor).

Exercise may be the centerpiece of all the countermeasures utilized inflight, both from the cardiovascular and musculoskeletal systems standpoints. Short, but intensive daily exercise, with proper hydration before and after each session, seems to be appropriate. Exercise should be divided into isotonic and isometric sessions, starting early in the mission, and coupled with a carefully controlled diet. Daily walking and running on a treadmill for up to one hour should provide enough protection for the cardiovascular and muscular systems. Appropriately designed exercise activities to maintain upper body muscle force and mass should also be used on a regular basis. There is a distinct need to establish a safe and efficacious means of rehydration prior to reentry, besides ingestion of normal saline. Consideration should be given to adding glucose and other electrolytes to the normal saline in order to facilitate absorption and retention fluids. Administration of plasma expanders might present added technical complexity, since they are primarily designed for intravenous routes. Drugs such as diphosphonates, vitamin D, calcium supplements, and anabolic hormones can also be utilized in the overall program of countermeasures, when gastrointestinal absorption rates and the overall metabolic pathways in weightlessness are better understood. A significant amount of basic research is required on the ground and in flight before adequate progress can be made in the area of countermeasure utilization.

Table 6
SPACE FLIGHT URINE BIOCHEMICAL RESULTS

Substance	Mission type	
	STS	Skylab
Potassium	▲	▲
Calcium	▲	▲
Phosphates	▲	▲
Citrate	No change*	?
Oxalate	No change*	?
Magnesium	▲	▲
Uric acid	+ or −	+ or −
Osmolality	▲	▲

†One crewmember on STS 61-C

REFERENCES

1. A.E. Nicogossian and J.F. Parker, *Space Physiology and Medicine* (NASA SP-447), pp. 165-185. U.S. Government Printing Office, Washington, D.C. (1977).

2. G.W. Hoffler, R.L. Johnston, A.E. Nicogossian, S.A. Bergmand and M.M. Jackson, Vectorcardiographic Results from Skylab Medical Experiment M092: Lower Body Negative Pressure. In *Biomedical Results from Skylab*, (Edited by R.S. Johnston and L.F. Dietlein), (NASA SP-377). U.S. Government Printing Office, Washington, D.C. (1977).

3. J.A. Rummel, C.F. Sawin, E.L. Michel, M.C. Buderer and W.T. Thornton, Exercise and long duration spaceflight through 84 days. *J.A.M.W.A.* 30, 173-187 (1975).

4. C.S. Leach, P.C. Johnson and W.W. Suki, Current concepts of space flight-induced changes. In *Hormonal Control of Fluid and Electrolyte Metabolism. The Physiologist* 26, 5-24 - 5-27 (1983).

HEALTH MAINTENANCE ON SPACE STATION

James S. Logan[*]

Space Station mission success is highly dependent on maintaining inflight crew health and safety. Medical support for extended manned missions must include capabilities for prevention, diagnosis, and therapy in all phases of the mission: pre-flight, inflight, and post-flight. Design and development of an adequate inflight health care delivery system, real time environment monitoring, physiological countermeasures, and medical rescue and recovery of all ill/injured crewmembers will present unique challenges to aerospace physicians, scientists, and engineers.

INTRODUCTION

As space exploration progresses toward longer duration missions, the role of life sciences and space medicine will undoubtedly expand. Medical care in space and the successful resolution of numerous biomedical problems relating to physiological adaptation to micro-G may lead the list of technologies and capabilities which could severely limit increasing mission duration for manned space flight. Unless a genuine attempt is made to solve current and anticipated problems in the biomedical area, mission planners will discover the human link in the chain may be the most vulnerable. Without a high priority sustained effort, significant biomedical issues will preclude the timely accomplishment of extended Space Station, lunar base, and/or manned mission to Mars.

In its broadest context, crew health maintenance encompasses the triad of modern medicine: prevention, diagnosis, and therapy. This approach applies equally to the crewmember and his/her environment and includes medical certification, crew selection, pre-flight health stabilization, inflight medical capabilities, physiological countermeasures, spacecraft environmental monitoring, contamination containment, control, and disposal, and rescue and recovery. Conventional medicine usually consists of an abnormal subject (i.e., patient) in a normal environment. Environmental medicine and occupational medicine usually consists of the interaction between a normal subject and an abnormal environment. Clinical space medicine presents the ultimate challenge: an abnormal subject in an abnormal environment. In addition, medical care in space must be accomplished with numerous operational constraints such as severely limited mass, volume, and power available for biomedical equipment. The physical isolation from the terrestrial medical infrastructure is a significant design drive for physicians and engineers.

The medical operations concept for Space Station consists of:

---

[*] M.D., Chief of Medical Operations, NASA Johnson Space Center, Houston, Texas 77058.

1. providing full service medical/dental care from the time a crewmember is selected;

2. utilizing pre-flight, inflight, and post-flight biomedical data recovery to support health care delivery and extend mission duration;

3. drastically improving inflight preventive, diagnostic, and treatment capability in selected areas;

4. the initiation, maintenance, and enhancement of a medically comprehensive environmental monitoring and control program;

5. providing an adequate rescue and recovery capability.

NASA medical operations has the responsibility to provide comprehensive medical/dental coverage and health maintenance from the time a crewmember is selected to be a professional astronaut or a non-astronaut slated to fly on a specific mission. NASA flight surgeons also have the authority to grant medical certification for space flight for all potential crewmembers. The certification exam is performed once a year. Only clinical findings and laboratory results obtained during that exam can be used to grant or not grant medical certification. All biomedical data obtained for research purposes (even operational research) cannot be used in the medical certification decision making process.

MEDICAL CERTIFICATION

The initial (Project Mercury) medical standards for astronaut selection, retention, and flight certification were rigid due to the hypothetical deleterious physiological effects (reversible and irreversible) of weightlessness. It was felt (given the lack of space flight experience at the time) that the micro-G environment would have a negative effect on physiological performance. Because the effects of space flight were not known, it was argued that the "baseline" should be as physiologically "normal" (i.e., free of all disease) as possible. As American space flight experience increased, it became apparent that the original medical selection standards were unnecessarily strict. Although rigid vision, hearing, and performance standards appeared justified for those astronauts having direct control of the vehicle, another class of crewmembers could perform their important mission functions while meeting less rigorous medical standards.

The tendency to permit more liberal medical selection and retention standards persisted into the STS program. The basic approach to medical selection standards for astronauts with the possible exception of Pilot (Class I) was to accept all candidates who (1) could perform an emergency egress; (2) could utilize standard equipment (i.e., space suits, launch and entry helmets, etc.); and (3) were free from acute and chronic disease which could either jeopardize a mission or a crewmember. Many chronic diseases can be adequately managed by modern therapeutical techniques (for example, high blood pressure). Therefore, the chronic use of medication could be granted a medical waiver by the Space Medicine Board. Pilot astronauts must still meet rigid visual and auditory standards.

For STS, there are four certification classes: (1) Class I (Pilot); (2) Class II (Mission Specialist); (3) Class II (Payload Specialist); and (4) Class IV (Citizen Observer). Class III and IV standards are the most liberal as these crewmembers are not career astronauts. The goal has been to open up opportunities for flight experience to the widest section of the population possible without compromising either the mission or personal safety.

Waivers can be granted on an individual basis if approved by the Space Medicine Board. Historically, there have been two trends regarding medical certification. The first is that each time medical standards have been revised, they have become more liberal. The second is that the older astronaut population and increased short duration flight experience have resulted in an increasing number of waivers.

The potential complexities of longer duration space flight may reverse the above trends to a degree. A condition which may not compromise a 10-day mission could significantly affect a 120-day mission. One conclusion is obvious: without adequate inflight medical capability, Station medical selection and retention standards will have to be much more conservative than STS standards. In addition, without inflight medical capabilities, the philosophy of medical waivers would require re-examination. Even with adequate inflight medical care capabilities, it seems prudent to make Station medication certification and retention standards more restrictive. The management of the medical risk must encompass both rational selection standards and adequate inflight medical care capabilities. Without adequate inflight medical capabilities and expertise, extremely rigid selection and retention standards would necessitate younger crews and shorter flight careers.

CREW SELECTION

Historically, the role of the NASA medical establishment has been to determine whether or not a potential crewmember meets all applicable medical standards. For STS, the actual selection of crewmembers for a specific mission remained a management function. Management has used a number of criteria to determine the mission specific skill mix of a crew. This tradition will probably continue into the Space Station era with minor modifications.

Crew selection for long-duration missions requires careful consideration of numerous complex issues which are not significant factors for short-duration missions. Unfortunately, these issues cannot be adequately quantified. The complex crew selection issues are best decided by close interaction and communication between the medical and flight operations communities. However, the operational medical establishment has initiated an ongoing program to quantify relevant psychological factors in crewmembers pre/post selection. The training of all potential crewmembers includes a basic and applied knowledge of interpersonal psychological transactional analysis) which can be easily utilized by the psychological non-professional. Management should have the option to remove any crewmember deemed an operational risk to the successful completion of the mission. Significant uncontrolled psychological deterioration in a crewmember due to the unique psychological/physical parameters of long-duration missions could pose a threat to the crewmember him/herself, other members of the crew, and the mission.

HEALTH STABILIZATION PROGRAM

Because of several inflight illnesses secondary to presumed exposure to prevailing infectious agents (most likely viruses) the week prior to flight during the Gemini and early Apollo flights, a Health Stabilization Program (HSP) was initiated after Apollo 7. The HSP was revised in 1982 for the STS program. The purpose of the program was to limit crew contact with people who may expose the crew to infectious agents having a short (4-7 day) incubation time. Limiting crew exposure the week prior to flight drastically reduced the incidence of inflight illness on STS flights due to common respiratory or flu-like infectious agents. A comparison of the incidences of inflight viral illness prior to and after initiation of a HSP demonstrated the STS HSP was effective at the P.05 statistical significance level.

The emphasis of HSP is prevention because inflight illnesses due to exposure prior to flight are preventable. The HSP is a "voluntary" program in the sense that the program only works well if all participants are cooperative and motivated. The seven-day time frame for STS takes care of the majority (but by no means all) of common prevailing infectious illnesses. The Station HSP may be lengthened to 14 days to cover the vast majority of viral illnesses.

The current HSP does not place the crew in "quarantine" or "isolation" in any sense. However, during the 14 days prior to a mission, crews are asked not to venture into crowded conditions (for example: movie theaters, restaurants/cafeterias, concert halls, etc.) and they are encourage to live (and eat) in specially designed and maintained crew facilities. Only those people designated as "primary contacts" (PCs) may come within six feet of a crewmember. Primary contact status can be conferred upon personnel having a need to interact with the crew by a physician after a brief exam and laboratory screen. PC status is good for one year but PCs are reminded that it is their responsibility to report to a NASA site physician, should they come down with an illness during the time HSP is in effect. The physician then makes a determination whether or not to rescind PC status for that individual.

Epidemiological studies of remote populations indicate an increased incidence of contagious illnesses when "newcomers" are introduced into a remote population. For example, when small groups of people winter over in Antarctica, they "pass around" various contagious illnesses early in the mission. (NOTE: crews chosen to winter over do not undergo a health stabilization-type program). After the first two weeks the incidence of infectious illness markedly decreases due to a decreasing population at risk. If, for some reason, a new person is introduced into the population, the previously isolated population is at risk for whatever new infectious agents the newcomer might bring with him/her. Therefore, a new round of illnesses sweep through the original "isolated" population. The station scenario may require change of only a portion of the crew during each STS visit. It is obvious that HSP is important not only for the original crew but for visiting crews as well.

INFLIGHT MEDICAL CAPABILITIES

Longer mission duration, larger crew size, and the lack of an immediate nominal return to Earth capability distinguish Space Station mission scenarios from STS operations. Although a medical kit is standard equipment for all STS flights, a moderate to severe medical contingency would require mission termination and deorbit to permit delivery of appropriate medical treatment on the ground. A similar approach to a Space Station medical contingency would be impractical (and most likely life threatening) due to the cost and time required to effect a medical "rescue". Initial estimates of the cost incurred for an unplanned STS mission for medical rescue (i.e., ambulance) range from 125-250 million dollars per rescue attempt. In addition, the time required to effect an STS rescue has been estimated to be in the range of 28-45 days. Therefore, the development of an adequate inflight health care delivery system is essential to Station mission success.

The Station inflight health care delivery system is designed to incorporate the triad of modern medicine: prevention, diagnosis, and therapy. Prevention includes routine health maintenance, the establishment of physiologic "norms", exercise countermeasures designed to prevent physiologic adaptation to the weightless state resulting in decreased cardiac and skeletal muscle performance, bone mineral loss and other deleterious effects. The medical facility will be linked to the environment monitoring system to ensure a biologically safe environment. Diagnosis requires the presence of physicians' instruments for performing a physical exam, an inflight laboratory with clinical chemistry, hematology (blood count), urine analysis, and microbiology capabilities, a radiographic and nonradiographic imaging system, and electrophysiologic monitoring. Therapy requires intravenous fluid production and administration, pharmacy, central supply, anesthesia, minor surgical/dental, medical life support, and mechanical ventilation capabilities. A hyperbaric treatment facility (modified airlock) is required for the treatment of altitude decompression sickness and air embolus. The entire medical facility will be integrated via a computer system compatible with the Station computer system for uplink/downlink of medical/biological parameters to ground medical personnel.

The equipment of the inflight health care delivery system is located at the Station Health Maintenance Facility (HMF). Additional medical equipment is located in Station "safe havens", should the module in which the HMF is located become nonfunctional. Much of the HMF equipment must be transportable to facilitate the rescue and return to Earth of an ill and/or injured patient. The HMF will be required to be fully operational at Permanent Manned Presence (PMP) or any Station mode other than STS attended operations.

The goal of the Health Maintenance Facility is to effectively provide inflight preventive, diagnostic, and therapeutic medical capabilities in accordance with U.S. clinically acceptable current and anticipated medical practice standards within the Space Station program constraints. There are five prime objectives of the inflight medical care system:

1. Ensure crew safety and health maintenance during routine operations;

91

2. Prevent excess mortality (death) and morbidity (illness/disease);

3. Prevent early mission termination due to medical contingency;

4. Prevent an unnecessary rescue;

5. Increase the probability of success of a necessary rescue.

There may be unavoidable inflight mortality and morbidity during the lifetime of the Station just as there is unavoidable mortality and morbidity in terrestrial settings (including major medical centers). However, many medical/surgical conditions can be definitively treated with minimal medical equipment and onboard medical expertise. Many other medical/surgical conditions can be managed over rather long periods of time enabling definitive treatment to be postponed to a later date. Adequate inflight medical capabilities decrease the risk of terminating a Station mission early due to medical concerns. Depending on the medical condition, a crewmember could be supported until the scheduled end of mission, thus preventing a costly rescue.

The addition of a Crew Emergency Rescue Vehicle (CERV) will impact the design of the HMF. The presence of a CERV will necessitate expanded inflight medical stabilization and treatment capabilities to enhance medical coverage.

Early in the program at least two Station crewmembers per mission will be selected, trained, and certified as a "Crew Medical Officer" (CMO). As a minimum, the CMOs will have the equivalent of Emergency Medical Technician (EMT) training. They will also undergo intense training on all HMF subsystems. The advantages of a physician crewmember is obvious. The single most effective means to maximize the inflight medical capabilities as a function of the weight and volume of the HMF is to assign a physician/surgeon to fly on every mission. Eventually HMF capabilities will be upgraded to include general surgery capability. A clinically current general surgeon could then be assigned to each crew. A physician/surgeon crewmember should be cross-trained to perform a multitude of other required Station and/or payload duties.

PHYSIOLOGIC COUNTERMEASURES

Sufficient long-duration inflight data do not exist to adequately justify a scientifically valid "exercise prescription" for Space Station. Exercise protocols must be utilized to prevent physiologic adaptation to the micro-G environment. Exercise can be thought of as a "drug" designed to minimize cardiovascular deconditioning, skeletal muscle deconditioning, and bone mineral loss. However, the "drug" must be administered in the correct "dose" and "frequency" of administration to maximize the efficacy of the "medication."

Cardiovascular deconditioning was first documented in 100% of the Gemini space crews. By the final Skylab mission (84 days), crews were exercising (aerobic exercise) 1.5 hours per day. Some of the long-duration Soviet crews have reported that exercise is scheduled for approximately 3.5 hours a day per crewmember, a length of time which most American missions planners found unacceptable.

From an operational perspective, the most important areas of physiologic deconditioning (in decreasing order of importance) are:

1. Cardiovascular deconditioning;

2. Skeletal muscle deconditioning;

3. Bone mineral loss.

The physiologic changes observed inflight actually represent biological adaptation to a new environment, analogous to the adaptation that occurs when moving into a hot or cold climate or one at altitude. The changes which occur in micro-G are not deleterious during nominal micro-G operations but become so if conditions require increased muscle strength or cardiac reserve. For example, the cardiovascular and skeletal muscle "adaptations" to micro-G are not, by themselves, dangerous. However, should a difficult contingency Extravehicular (EVA) or Intravehicular (IVA) Activity become necessary requiring increased muscle strength and cardiac reserve, crew performance could be significantly affected.

Cardiovascular deconditioning requires aerobic (high frequency, low maintenance) exercise. A treadmill, bicycle ergometer, and/or rowing machine may be provided as inflight exercise devices. Skeletal muscle deconditioning requires strength and intensity exercise (low frequency, high resistance). For this reason, several force generators are being developed to exercise major muscle groups. All exercise devices must be fully instrumented, so that exercise profiles and associated physiologic data (mostly heart rate) can be downlinked to physicians on the ground. In addition, every 2-3 weeks each crewmember may undergo a submaximal stress test to fully quantify cardiac reserve. Utilizing this approach, physicians could track the rate of deconditioning for a specific crewmember and intervene to change the exercise "prescription" if necessary. A physiologically disastrous EVA or contingency immediately post-flight is not the time to discover that the exercise prescription is not working.

Each exercise device will probably be linked to an immediate physiological feedback display and/or a interactive motivational program using graphics and/or complex video sequences. Crewmembers may also have the choice of reading text, watching TV, or looking out the window during the exercise period. One of the highest priorities is to make the daily exercise period as enjoyable as possible. Crewmembers must have a certain amount of flexibility in determining their own exercise program within operationally accepted limits of deconditioning.

The question of bone demineralization has received much attention. Pre/post-flight bone density measurements will be obtained on every Station crewmember. An intense research effort will be initiated to determine whether or not the bone mineral lost during micro-G exposure is replenished post-flight. Another very important area of operational research will be the verification of the time required between long-duration missions to permit return of all physiologic subsystems to pre-flight conditioning levels.

ENVIRONMENTAL MONITORING

The difference between process control for any spacecraft environmental control and life support system (ECLSS) and true environmental monitoring is often not appreciated. Process control implies measurement of the composition and "purity" of the output of the Environmental Control and Life Support System (ECLSS), usually spacecraft atmosphere and potable water. Process control is an essential element of the ECLSS but exists only to verify that the output of a system meets the specifications for which the system was designed.

Environmental Monitoring (EM), on the other hand, seeks to quantify and track all potential biological hazards within an environment. The philosophy for EM is the measurement of the total biohazard. For example, ECLSS process determines whether the system is delivering a sea level atmosphere consisting of 80% nitrogen and 20% oxygen. EM seeks to measure all volatile substances (organic and inorganic), particulate matter, and the microbial load (bacteria, fungi, etc.) of air that is breathed by crewmembers. In addition, the microbial load of spacecraft surfaces is also measured. Even the microbial load of individual crewmember's ear canals, nasal passages, and skin can be measured.

On short-duration STS missions, environmental monitoring is accomplished pre-flight, inflight, and post-flight. Numerous samples of the spacecraft environment are taken several times prior to flight and immediately post-flight to attempt to determine the mechanisms of environmental contamination. Numerous inflight samples of air are taken for post-flight analysis to quantify the increase of particulate matter and volatile substances as a function of mission duration and crew size. Inflight samples of water have also been obtained on several missions for post-flight analysis.

Because STS missions are of short duration and the vehicle is returned to Earth for thorough cleaning after every mission, there is no justifiable requirement for real time environmental monitoring. However, pre-flight, post-flight, and ground analysis of samples obtained inflight has identified some disturbing trends which are directly applicable to Station.

An orbiter's maiden voyage is the dirtiest for the atmosphere. The cabin atmosphere was so filled with particulate matter from the size of dust to small bolts on Discovery's maiden voyage (41-D), the crew reported the "flashlight beam" effect when sunlight came in through the windows. Massive amounts of particulate matter floating in the cabin were obtained in small sample bags by the crew and returned to Earth. These particulates can pose a health threat (corneal injury, inhalation or ingestion of large particulate matter) in addition to the potential of damaging sensitive avionic equipment either by direct interference or blocking essential pathways for air cooling. After the maiden voyage, particulates become less of a problem to repeat short duration missions. However, the measured particulates increase as a function of mission duration and crew size. In the Skylab program, the first crew reported increased particulates but with time particulates decreased, indicating that the capacity of the Skylab ECLSS system to filter the atmosphere exceeded STS capacity.

The microbial load of the shuttle increases directly as a function of mission duration and crew size. Detailed microbial examinations of returning crewmembers demonstrate transfer of potential pathogens from one crewmember to others. Although initially not confirmed, the data (in vitro mitogen stimulation studies of circulating lymphocytes obtained immediately post-flight) suggest depressed immune system function following even short duration exposure to micro-G. Assessing immune function will become a high priority on longer duration missions. Between missions, the orbiter crew compartments are scrubbed down with a disinfectant solution including an organic solvent designed to dissolve bacterial and fungal cell walls. Such solutions can not be used in a closed station environment due to crew exposure concerns. Therefore, the EM program must develop safe and effective procedures to clean and disinfect spacecraft surfaces (including the inner EMU surfaces) inflight. The disinfectant solutions developed for Space Station must be non-toxic to humans.

On the first Skylab mission, a sunshield failed to deploy resulting in significant heating of the spacecraft cabin. Although the crew carried a crude air sampler with them to "sniff" the air abroad Skylab before leaving the command module after docking, the crew themselves were the "dosimeters" to measure possible contamination. The presence of inflight activities such as materials processing will greatly magnify the problem of real time contamination monitoring, containment, and control on Station. Multiple high-temperature materials processing furnaces will produce a myriad of potentially dangerous substances.

There have been concerns during Space Station design that the Station could become an example of runaway "tight building syndrome". Because of the energy efficiency requirements of terrestrial commercial and residential buildings constructed after the oil embargoes of the 1970s, a new toxicological phenomenon of "tight building syndrome" was identified. Workers were found to be suffering acute and chronic effects of toxic exposure. When air samples were obtained from these buildings, the levels of many toxic substances were found to be significantly above industrial OSHA and NIOSH standards. These findings, discovered mostly in office buildings, surprised many experts in the occupational health and safety disciplines. The buildings were so efficient that air was not being replaced at a rate that kept up with the accumulation of toxic substances. In many major cities, the air inside certain office buildings was worse than the air outside. The "tight building syndrome" may prove applicable to the Station. Without real time air sampling and monitoring, the Station could become a runaway example of tight building syndrome possibly requiring crew evacuation due to health concerns.

There are also concerns regarding the potential microbial load of the Station. The Station may have to be completely disinfected and cleaned, module by module, rack by rack, at some frequency to be determined. Fungi may grow especially well on filters and grids protecting sensitive avionic equipment. The first indications of greater than expected fungal growth could be thermal overtemp warnings from equipment bays, as fungal growth on grids and filters may be responsible for decreased cooling by air flow.

The disposal of various relatively nontoxic materials (using common plumbing for disposal) could result in episodic contamination on Station. The residue of two or more relatively inert substances could react with each other in the waste disposal plumbing resulting in the formation of moderately toxic compounds in significant doses. On the ground such materials interaction problems are solved by sequential disposal, a process by which a massive amount of a dilutant (usually water) is used to wash away any residual substance in the disposal plumbing system before disposal of a second substance. However, materials interaction difficulties have been reported in several incidents involving submarines. Disposal procedures using massive dilutants are obviously impractical for Station. The lack of adequate planning in the design phase of Station could result in curtailed materials processing operations.

In spite of stringent safety and materials isolation requirements, there will always be the possibility of a toxic "spill" or toxic "incidents" on the Station. Adequate procedures and equipment for contamination isolation, containment, control, and cleanup must be developed.

The environmental monitoring systems will be linked to the Station Health Maintenance Facility computer system. the information will be downlinked to physicians and environmental specialists on the ground for analysis. The environmental monitoring issues have the real potential of being a Station "show stopper".

RESCUE AND RECOVERY

At least three scenarios requiring a Crew Emergency Rescue Vehicle (CERV) have been identified: (1) grounded STS; (2) Space Station emergency; and (3) inflight medical contingency.

In the event STS orbiters are unavailable (for a significant amount of time) for re-supply and servicing of the Station (such as a 51-L type disaster occurring on a Station re-supply mission), a CERV could be the only option for crew return to Earth. CERV capability has special merit if the extended mission duration required by the contingency exceeded onboard consumable reserves. If indicated, CERV return of a portion of the crew could extend the stay time of a smaller group of Station crewmembers.

A Station contingency such as the loss of power, fire, toxic exposure, loss of atmosphere, or other catastrophic problem could necessitate immediate evacuation and/or return of some or all crewmembers to Earth. It is likely any scenario requiring evacuation might also involve a medical problem. Some situations might permit a safe return to the Station after a short period of time. In this scenario, the CERV could be used as a "lifeboat" until Station systems are "safed". For example, an accident causing an acute toxic exposure could be resolved (with assistance from ground controllers) over a 24-48 hour period, thus permitting return of the crew.

A significant inflight medical contingency would also be a candidate for CERV rescue. Of the three scenarios, medical rescue is probably the most likely. It seems unlikely that a severely ill or injured crewmember would be allowed to perish on the Station if a CERV were available. Therefore, the mere presence of a CERV on Station may create an obligation to use it, if necessary, to save the life of a crewmember. However, a CERV, if implemented, should be designed to satisfy certain medical transport requirements.

The presence of a CERV would also serve as a driver to enhance rather than reduce inflight medical capabilities. CERV options would not alter the preventive capabilities of the HMF. Inflight diagnostic capabilities will be essential to the process of deciding when and when not to utilize a CERV. If CERV capability is realized, intensive resuscitation and patient stabilization (i.e., treatment) capabilities will be required to ready the patient for transport, otherwise the transport itself may be more dangerous to the patient than the expected clinical outcome of the condition if immediate rescue were not possible.

An example of CERV driven enhancement of HMF functions is the concept of inflight blood banking: frozen storage of crew cross-matched blood products with on-board capabilities to thaw, process (wash), and safely administer such products to crewmembers. Without CERV capability, blood banking is considered impractical from a weight and volume standpoint. The majority of conditions encountered on Station requiring the administration of blood products would most likely be candidates for surgical intervention. If definitive therapy in the form of general surgery is not possible (general surgery capability is not planned for the initial years of Station), the chances of being able to keep up with a crewmember's blood loss for more than a few hours is low. However, if immediate or short-term transport is a possibility, the medical emphasis should be on stabilization and transport, in which case the ability to administer blood products could be a lifesaving procedure.

The decision to utilize a CERV for medical contingencies would necessitate an evaluation of the seriousness of the illness, its prognosis, and a real time analysis of the benefit versus risk of CERV transport for the affected crewmembers. Part of the risk versus benefit analysis will depend on the type of CERV (i.e., entry profile) and the length of time from splash down to arrival at a definitive medical care facility.

The higher the magnitude and duration of G forces experienced on entry, the greater the medical risk for transport of severely ill or injured crewmembers. Physiological tolerance to G forces is greatest in the +Gx direction ("eye balls in", accelerative force from the chest to back). For instance, there are a variety of medical conditions which precluded a DC-9 (standard USAF MEDEVAC transport jet) takeoff due to unacceptable acceleration effects. Although there are no studies to document the effects of acceleration on transport of critically ill patients, there are studies which show decreased tolerance to acceleration by normal subjects after short periods of deconditioning. It is assumed even "healthy" crewmembers would be impaired to a degree during and immediately after entry, especially after longer duration missions. It seems rational to conclude, based on terrestrial experience with the effects of minor stress (for example a change of position from supine to sitting) in ill or injured patients, acceleration effects would be greatly magnified in medically compromised crewmembers. High-G vehicle designs are therefore unacceptable for the vast majority of conditions requiring medical transport. Other potential acceleration (or deceleration) effects of CERV entry (spin stabilization, landing impact) must be kept to a minimum for similar reasons.

Another significant factor in the risk versus benefit decision to return an ill or injured crewmember via CERV is the length of time between splashdown and arrival at a definitive medical care facility. From a medical perspective, it would make little sense to transport a medically compromised crewmember from a stable environment with sophisticated medical facilities (Space Station with an HMF) to a dynamic environment (i.e., entry and landing via CERV) with little or no immediately available medical facilities. (NOTE: an aircraft carrier does not satisfy the definition of a definitive medical care facility).

The transport of an ill or injured crewmember from the Station to the middle of the Indian, Pacific, or Atlantic ocean, hours from pickup and hundreds of miles from a definitive medical care facility, should be avoided. Agency management must be made to realize such a scenario could literally be a "death sentence" for a medically compromised crewmember. To maximize coverage for the medical risk, the Station HMF, the inflight medical expertise, the CERV/entry profile, and the make-up of rescue and recovery forces should be synergistically designed and integrated.

One current option for operational medical rescue and recovery consists of two CERVs (Apollo style capsules outfitted for 6 crewmembers). Each CERV would have the capability for accommodating at least one injured or ill crewmember (i.e., special restraints, seat with litter capability and impact attenuation, egress assistance, etc.). There would be a stowage space for specific medical equipment and supplies (i.e., a basic survival/first-aid kit for post landing). Several small pieces of transportable (stored at HMF) medical life support equipment could be attached to the litter (i.e., cardiac monitor and defibrillator, small ventilator, etc.).

The entry profile would not exceed 3 Gs with accelerative forces only in the +Gz axis (eye balls in). High rate spin stabilization would not be required. The CERV would have the capability to loiter in orbit for up to eight hours to permit an entry trajectory with a landing footprint within 100 miles of a coastal definitive medical care facility and dedicated search and rescue (SAR) forces. After touchdown, crew pick-up by trained SAR forces would be accomplished within 90 minutes. After pick-up, transfer to a definitive medical care facility would occur within two hours.

The utilization of a CERV for medical transport would be a real time decision by the crew medical officer(s), crew commander, ground-based medical personnel, station flight director(s), and NASA senior management. It is assumed that NASA management would not permit a crewmember to languish in orbit if any CERV capability were available. However, management should understand and accept the extremely high risk of returning a significantly compromised crewmember using an entry/recovery scenario not designed for medical transport and treatment.

CONCLUSION

The Medical Operations concept for Station incorporates clinical medical/dental care and health maintenance on the ground and in orbit. The biomedical aspects of long-duration space flight are complex and interdisciplinary. The successful resolution of biomedical issues and concerns requires the cooperation and active support of crewmembers, NASA medical personnel, managers, engineers, and life scientists. An ever increasing role for life science is essential to continue manned exploration of the solar system.

CONSIDERATION FOR SOLAR SYSTEM EXPLORATION: A SYSTEM TO MARS[*]

Arnauld.E. Nicogossian[†] and Victoria Garshnek[‡]

A piloted mission to Mars will challenge the human capacity to live and work in extreme environments for an extended period of time. Medical specialists will be called upon to certify that individuals selected for such a voyage are healthy enough to undergo 2 to 3 years of space flight. Spacecraft life support systems must prevent accumulation of toxic chemicals; psychological issues (isolation, confinement) will acquire greater importance; and radiation exposures could exceed Apollo mission doses by orders of magnitude. Other critical issues that must be addressed include cardiovascular and musculoskeletal deconditioning, immunological and hematological changes, and nutritional considerations. Partial prevention of physiological adaptation to weightlessness through various countermeasures geared to the musculoskeletal and cardiovascular systems seems a natural approach to successful readaptation to Earth's gravity. However, doubts arise as to the efficacy of these countermeasures given the extended time required for a round trip to Mars. Readjustment to Earth's gravity may be quite difficult after such a voyage. Should physiological countermeasures prove insufficient, some level of artificial gravity may need to be provided. All of these issues must be better understood and resolved to guarantee productive human exploration of the Martian surface, and safe readaptation upon return to Earth.

INTRODUCTION

Experience has shown that humans can live and work in space for periods approaching one year. However, even short excursions into near-Earth orbit or to the moon have indicated that there is a penalty to be paid upon return to Earth's gravity field once adaptation to weightlessness has taken place. Even though a reduced gravity field exists on Mars, long-duration space travel in excess of one year to this less hospitable planet will challenge the resources of the medical knowledge base.

Before humans can safely undertake a flight to Mars--and safely return--certain stressors inherent to space flight and their physiological and psychological consequences must be considered. These stressors include altered gravitational loads

*   Reprinted with permission of Nihon University, 8-24, Kudan-Minami 4-chome, Chiyoda-ku, Tokyo 102, Japan, from Proceedings of NISAS '87 (Nihon University Research Institute, Dec. 5-9, 1987).

†   M.D., Life Sciences Division, NASA Headquarters, 600 Independence Ave., S.W., Washington, D.C. 20546.

‡   Ph.D., The George Washington University, Science Communications Studies, Washington, D.C. 20006.

(launch, weightlessness, reentry), sustained workloads, cabin environment (possible toxicological events, confinement), and radiation.

The biomedical issues which need to be adequately understood are changes which occur in different body systems such as cardiovascular, immunological, hematological, and musculoskeletal systems. Other important issues include nutritional considerations and countermeasure development. In addition, appropriate medical selection, screening, and certification of crews must be done for the long mission. A facility for medical care and health maintenance, equipped with the necessary instrumentation and medications, should be provided on board the Mars transit and landing vehicles.

BIOMEDICAL ISSUES

Cardiovascular Deconditioning

The etiology of flight-induced cardiovascular deconditioning begins with a fluid shift of 1.5L to 2L from the lower to upper body. To accommodate this fluid redistribution a number of physiological readjustments occur. The first are probably an increased diuresis and decreased thirst as the cardiovascular system attempts to establish a new stable pressure/volume relationship. However, neither of these mechanisms have been definitely demonstrated during weightless space flight. The fluid shift actually begins before takeoff while the crew is supine in the spacecraft for hours in preparation for launch. The cardiovascular system reaches a point of stasis (usually within 36 hours). The size of the heart has been observed to decrease as a result of space flight (Ref. 1,2) and its electrical and mechanical activities indicate depressed function (decreased filling volume) (Ref. 2). These changes may increase the propensity for electrical instabilities and arrhythmias during EVA or after long duration missions; however, such data have not been statistically validated.

Return to Earth reverses the adaptive process, placing a gravitational stress on the cardiovascular system. Heart rate increases to maintain cardiac output, blood pooling occurs in the lower extremities, and the lower circulating fluid volume results in decreased cerebral blood flow and diminished orthostatic tolerance. Normal saline loading 4 hours before landing has been used as a countermeasure against orthostatic intolerance in the Space Shuttle Program. However, 4-day missions seem to be the optimum duration for use of this countermeasure whereas, for a 10-day mission, saline loading alone might be insufficient (Ref. 2). Therefore, factors other than hydrostatic pressure and fluid volume are probably involved (possibly muscle atrophy, nervous control, and resetting of baroreceptors). A somewhat modified protocol is implemented in conjunction with a Lower Body Negative Pressure (LBNP) device on Soviet long duration missions. How far cardiovascular changes would progress during a 2-3 year mission to Mars--and whether the cardiovascular system would regain "normal" function upon return to Earth--remain pressing questions.

Hematological/Immunological Changes

Accompanying the fluid shifts and the resulting decrease in plasma volume is the "space anemia" that has been observed consistently following manned space flights. Losses of red cell mass by U.S. astronauts have averaged 10-15%, accompanied by decreases in hemoglobin mass (12-33%) and losses in plasma volume (4-16%) (Ref. 3,4,5). Based on postflight estimates of total hemoglobin, Soviet cosmonauts in space missions lasting from 1-7 months have exhibited somewhat greater losses (Ref. 6). Restoration of red blood cell mass requires from 4-6 weeks following return to Earth, regardless of duration of space flight.

There are no reports suggesting that "space anemia" has had a clinical impact on the health and performance of crewmembers inflight or postflight. Nevertheless, inflight illness, injuries (loss of blood, hemorrhage), or life support malfunctions (hypoxic conditions) could possibly alter cardiovascular-respiratory requirements, further compromising the health status. Moreover, uncertainties exist as to the responses of the hematopoietic system during long-duration missions lasting a year or longer. Therefore, loss of red cell mass represents an operational medical problem in need of further investigation, especially in the areas of blood storage, blood substitutes, and transfusions.

No instances of inflight or postflight illnesses have been linked to alteration of cellular immune function; however, neutrophilia, relative lymphopenia, and a diminished blastogenic responsiveness of T-lymphocytes in postflight blood samples from astronauts and cosmonauts have been repeatedly observed, reverting to preflight values approximately 1 week postflight (Ref. 7,8,9,10,11,12,13). Other space-related alterations of immune function include postflight eosinopenia (Ref. 13), monocytopenia, reduced percentage of B-lymphocytes, decreased natural killer cell activity (Ref. 8), and production of a-interferon by lymphocytes (Ref. 14). The causes and mechanisms involved in these responses are not known, nor is it known at which stages of flight these responses occur.

Of concern here is the question of the immune system's ability to respond to stressors upon reaching another environment or returning to Earth. If further experience demonstrates that space flight does compromise immunocompetence, methods of effective intervention should be developed to decrease the probability that space crews in future long-duration missions would experience clinically significant immune dysfunction (Ref. 15)

Bone Changes

Another effect of microgravity is the loss of bone mass. Calcium losses have been estimated through carefully executed metabolic balance studies. Fecal and urinary calcium excretion were measured on Gemini, Apollo, and Skylab missions, and serum calcium levels were measured preflight and postflight. While mean urine calcium content continued to increase rapidly after takeoff, it reached a plateau within 30 days. In contrast, mean fecal calcium continued to increase steadily throughout flight (Ref. 16). Measurements made upon return to Earth indicated that urine calcium content had usually been reduced to preflight levels by the 10th day after landing, but fecal calcium was not reduced until the 20th postflight day.

The amount of calcium in the urine of Skylab astronauts increased by 60 to 100%, indirectly reflecting an overall bone loss of nearly half a percent per month-- even when the astronauts exercised vigorously. The critical question is whether these losses would continue unchecked throughout a long mission. If they persist, the consequences would eventually become serious. Once bones lose 20-25% of their mineral content, individual bones (particularly those in the legs and spine) would become fragile. If fractures occurred, would the lack of gravity impede proper healing? Without gravity, it is not clear whether proper healing would take place (Ref. 17).

Another problem involves the possibility of kidney stones forming out of calcium-saturated urine. Once formed, renal stones can be incapacitating. Even if they are excreted, recurrences are likely, which can also result in blockage of the ureter. An additional concern associated with hypercalciuria and proteinuria, especially in a closed and confined spacecraft with difficult hygiene conditions, will be the development of urinary system infections.

If, after return to Earth from a Mars mission, the body's calcium balance is restored before the bones have replaced the lost minerals, permanent bone damage could result. Therefore, the possibility that such long periods in microgravity might produce irreversible bone loss remains an important and crucial question.

Muscle Changes

Muscle studies have closely paralleled bone studies, relying heavily on comparisons of preflight and postflight measurements of muscle girth and strength. A reduction in both has been demonstrated postflight. Biomedical observations of crewmembers involved in the Gemini, Apollo, and Skylab missions revealed a decrease in exercise tolerance postflight. Strength testing following Skylab missions showed a decrease in arm extensor strength in 8 of 9 crewmen and a postflight decrease in leg extension force in all 9 crewmen (Ref. 18). There is no evidence that loss of muscle strength has operationally impacted any mission thus far, although a potential may exist for decreased performance during prolonged EVA on the Martian surface.

Analyses of serum drawn before and after space flight have shown a postflight increase in circulating nitrogen and creatinine kinase (indicating muscle breakdown) (Ref. 19). The muscle loss observed during space flight is probably accompanied by a conversion of muscle type. Analyses of rat muscle preflight and postfight indicated an increase in the amount of fast-twitch, or white muscle fiber, relative to the bulkier slow-twitch, or red muscle fiber (important in endurance exercise and posture) (Ref. 20). This type of fiber conversion has yet to be observed in humans.

Nutritional Considerations

A manned Mars mission will place greater demands on oxygen, water, and food supplies. If an open system is to be used, a large supply of these essential commodities will be necessary. Few data exist to judge whether the quantities of nutrients provided meet the metabolic needs during long-term flights; the results of the Skylab missions suggest that deficits may exist. Both the Skylab and Soviet experiences with diet have been in the form of "real foods" produced on Earth. If, for long-term flights, that approach is to be supplemented or replaced by a bioregenerative food system, then it will be essential to show that such a system would be equivalent in meeting the astronaut's energy and nutritive requirements (Ref. 21).

Caution must also be taken in the proper proportions of foods and supplements consumed by the crew. For example, diets high in animal protein and calcium combined with vigorous exercise (which further contributes to negative fluid balance and increased urine osmolality), coupled with unabated calcium excretion, can promote the development of renal calculi (Ref. 22).

Experiments to determine the nutritional and life support requirements for a trip to Mars will probably be performed on the Space Station. Therefore, it will be necessary to obtain detailed information on the nature of energy metabolism in space and its associated nutrient requirements over the long term.

Physiological Countermeasure Development

The musculoskeletal system has been of great concern to the Soviets, who have flown missions of up to 326 days. To counteract bone demineralization and muscle atrophy, Soviet space scientists have pursued certain countermeasures. For example, the Soviet "Penguin" suit places an axial load on the musculoskeletal system, requiring its wearer to work against the load to maintain an upright posture. Cosmonauts wear the suit during the waking hours, during which time they continuously work against the pull of the suit (Ref. 23). The suits are cumbersome and somewhat uncomfortable, therefore a question exists as to their practicality for a three-year journey. Cosmonauts also perform a regimen of onboard exercises, divided into 2 sessions and on 3-day cycles. Currently, they perform about 2 to 3 hours of exercise per day. Although exercise may be somewhat beneficial in slowing the rate of bone and muscle atrophy, after using the treadmill and bicycle ergometer, crews still return deconditioned.

The problem of postflight orthostatic intolerance is especially apparent in crews returning from long-duration space flight. Attempts to prevent or control cardiovascular deconditioning have involved inflight, reentry and postflight measures. These include vigorous, regularly scheduled exercise, repeated LBNP, and pre-reentry fluid and electrolyte replacement. In spite of variable and sometimes contradictory results obtained from studies of cardiovascular countermeasures, certain approaches have appeared promising to warrant further study and development. Among these are exercise (dynamic and static), prolonged LBNP stressing combined with oral replacement of fluids, and the use of anti-g suits (Ref. 24).

Partial prevention of physiological adaptation to weightlessness through various countermeasures geared to the musculoskeletal and cardiovascular systems seems a natural approach to successful readaptation to 1-g. But how effective will these countermeasures be for a flight to Mars and back? How difficult will readjustment to Earth's gravity be after such a voyage? If physiological countermeasures are not sufficient, some level of artificial gravity may have to be provided.

A feasible approach to producing artificial gravity for a mission to Mars would be to spin or rotate the spacecraft. A rotating spacecraft could be beneficial in alleviating the cardiovascular and musculoskeletal problems associated with microgravity. However, providing artificial gravity in this manner may have certain undesirable effects on the vestibular system. These are due mostly to complex Coriolis forces, which may introduce a difficult sensory-motor adjustment for crewmembers. A rotating environment might also cause a crewmember to become disoriented. For example, if he walks laterally to the rotation, two forces act upon him and the effect of the Coriolis force is worse. If the gravitation produced falls below 0.1-g, the crewmember will lose the traction needed for walking. Much early research needs to be done on the Space Station if a commitment is to be made either to a tether function or a rotating vehicle to produce artificial gravity. Critical experiments also need to be performed in space to determine the level of gravity (duration and fraction of) that will be needed to maintain the proper level of body fitness (Ref. 25).

ENVIRONMENTAL CONSIDERATIONS

Radiation

A central issue in manned space flight is the danger to the safety and health of humans posed by the ionizing radiation environment during long-term missions in space. In deep space the radiation environment is primarily galactic cosmic rays, which are composed of protons, alpha particles, and HZEs (energetic nuclei of heavy particles). Cosmic rays are very difficult to protect against. It is the geometry of exposure, not the intensity, that determines the biological effect of a cosmic particle. Particle acceleration experiments have shown that HZEs operate by single-hit kinetics: a particle strikes a target cell and its severity is determined by its position on the body and the angle at which the particle strikes the cell. During a 3-year round trip to Mars, the expected dose behind 2 1/2 grams per square centimeter shielding would be about 140 rem to the blood-forming organs (Ref. 26). This is substantial but still below the lifetime limit set by the NCRP. It is also higher than it need be, as the dose received on the Martian surface would be halved by the shielding effect of the planet's mass. Of great concern, however, is that such exposure to the heavy ion component of galactic cosmic radiation dominates the radiation dose equivalent for cancer induction.

The other important source of energetic particles is solar flares. Solar flares are intense, erratic bursts of proton radiation that tend to occur at 11-year intervals and deliver very high doses over short periods (a few hours or days). Without shielding, exposure to anomalously large events would be fatal to astronauts. But solar particle energies are much less than galactic cosmic rays, and they are stopped by less shielding material. The most likely solution to the problem would be to equip any long-range spacecraft or extraterrestrial habitat with a storm shelter. Such storm shelters can be made more efficient by using the water produced on board as a source of shielding. In addition, adequate solar flare early warning systems and biological dosimeters will need to be installed on the spacecraft. On the Martian surface, radiation exposure can be minimized by selecting sites protected by elevated terrain such as ravines, and by covering habitats with protective layers of Martian soil.

Cabin Environment/Toxicology

Safeguards against toxic chemical exposure during piloted missions to Mars will be extremely important for the management of crew health. The spacecraft cabin is a closed environment with a number of materials slowly releasing volatile components into the atmosphere which are potentially toxic. Unlike astronauts in near-Earth orbit, crewmembers on a Mars flight will be unable to remove themselves from the cabin during a toxic event. Therefore, the introduction of any toxic material into the atmosphere of such a closed system could have significant consequences, especially when considering the 9 or 10 months' transit time required for a Mars mission.

Potential sources of toxicity include offgassing of interior materials, thermal radiation or combustion of materials, and escape of chemicals from containers. Certain aspects of the mission could also influence the physiological severity of a toxic event. These include: mission duration, simultaneous exposure to other contaminants, deconditioning of crewmembers after long periods of sojourn in space, and simultaneous exposure to ionizing radiation.

The probability of significant toxic events can be reduced through proper material selection, ensuring heat stability of materials, proper containment of toxic chemicals, use of an alarm system to warn of toxic release into the atmosphere, protective clothing, the use of fume hoods while handling toxic chemicals, and the availability of refuge shelters for crewmembers in the event of high levels of toxic chemical contamination of the crew's immediate living environment. Also important are the availability of adequate provisions for periodic purging of the atmosphere and air revitalization systems. New SMAC limits will need to be established for potential containment of toxins. In addition, atmospheric contamination levels in the transit vehicle and lander will need to be monitored with a real-time analyzer (Ref. 27).

PERFORMANCE, BEHAVIOR, AND HUMAN FACTORS

Due to limited experience (in terms of the number of participants in long-term space missions), reliable predictive data are not available for predicting the likelihood of significant performance degradation and possible adverse behavioral effects during a long-term space flight to Mars involving multiple crewmembers.

Several factors in the environment of the Mars transit vehicle may become psychologically stressful, as the mission progresses from days to weeks to months. Examples of such factors are physical isolation, social deprivation, confinement, possible hazardous incidents (or the potential for their occurrence), lack of privacy, artificial life support, weightlessness (or, if the spacecraft is rotated to produce artificial gravity, the sensory discomfort involved in learning to live in a rotating environment).

Among the unresolved problems concerning the human components of the piloted Mars mission system are questions of optimal psychophysiological and psychological criteria and methods for crew selection, psychological and psychosocial factors in crew compatibility and productivity, and the effects of the spacecraft cabin environment on perceptual intellectual and motor skills. In addition, a great deal of basic research is still needed to provide an adequate data base for human factors applications in terms of perceptual, cognitive and psychomotor processes, capabilities, limitations in relation to spacecraft and space systems, spacecraft habitability, and interfaces between human operator and his equipment (Ref. 28).

MEDICAL ISSUES

Medical Selection/Disease Prediction

Mars transit and surface occupation create an unprecedented state of crew isolation, with no immediate return capability to Earth. For the duration of the trip, the crew will not have access to health care support of the same standards available on Earth. Medical screening of the crew will certainly need to be more extensive than for any previous mission. Space flight experience, however, has demonstrated that medical problems are relatively infrequent among properly screened individuals (Ref. 27).

To ensure that an individual will remain healthy to perform his designated duties during a Mars mission, it is desirable that long-term health prediction techniques be developed, since previously undiagnosed illnesses (e.g. malignancies) may become clinically significant during the course of a Martian voyage.

Health Maintenance

A greater portion of the resources allocated to health maintenance will most likely address the long-term medical monitoring of the crew and the practice of preventive medical techniques, such as exercise. The transit facility will need to provide appropriate hardware and techniques that will function in microgravity (in an emergency mode, even if artificial gravity is provided). The 1/3-g on the Martian surface will simplify some procedures, such as surgery, that would otherwise be difficult to perform in microgravity.

CONCLUSION

A manned mission to Mars will challenge the human capacity to live and work in extreme environments for an extended period of time. Never before has medicine been called upon to ensure that an individual will remain healthy enough to perform designated duties for 2 years following an examination. There is every reason to believe that mankind will be capable of launching a manned mission to Mars in the future. At the present time, important questions must be answered regarding physiological effects of microgravity, the need for artificial gravity, radiation, psychological stress, nutrition, life support, and the provision of necessary medical facilities and care. The problem at hand is not that humans are too fragile to pursue a mission to Mars or colonize the planet at some point in the future, but that we should direct our efforts and ingenuity toward providing the necessary conditions and protection that will enable humans to survive the voyage, work effectively on the Martian surface, return safely to Earth, and readjust to terrestrial conditions.

REFERENCES

1. Nicogossian, A.E., Hoffler, G.W., Johnson, R.L., and Gowen, R.J. "Determination of cardiac size following space missions of different durations: The second manned Skylab mission". *Aviat. Space and Environ. Med.,* 47(4): 362-365, 1976.

2. Bungo, M.W., Bagian, T.M., Bowman, M.A., and Levitan, B.M. (Eds.). "Results of the Life Sciences Detailed Supplementary Objectives (DSOs) Conducted Aboard the Space Shuttle From 1981 to 1986". *NASA TM-58280,* 1987.

3. Cogoli, A. "Hematological and Immunological Changes During Space Flight". *Acta Astronautica,* 8: 995-1002, 1981.

4. Johnson, P.C. "The Erythropoietic Effects of Weightlessness". In: *Current Concepts in Erythropoiesis* (G.D.R. Dunn, Ed.). John Wiley and Sons, New York, p. 279-300, 1983.

5. Kimzey, S.L. "A Review of Hematology Studies Associated With Space Flight". *Biorheology,* 16: 13-21, 1979.

6. Gazenko, O.G. "Investigations in Outer Space Conducted During 1982". *Aviat. Space Environ. Med.,* 54: 949-951, 1983.

7. Barone, R.P. and Caren, L.D. "The Immune System: Effects of Hypergravity and Hypogravity". *Aviat. Space Environ. Med.,* 55: 1063-1068, 1984.

8. Cogoli, A. and Tschopp, A. "Lymphocyte Reactivity During Space Flight". *Immunol. Today* 6: 1-4, 1985.

9. Kimzey, S.L., Fischer, C.L., Johnson, P.C., Ritzmann, S.E., and Mengel, C.E. "Hematology and Immunology Studies". In: *Biomedical Results of Apollo,* (R.S. Johnston, L.F. Dietlein, and C.A. Berry, Eds.). *NASA SP-368,* NASA, Washington, D.C., p. 197-226, 1975a.

10. Kimzey, S.L., Ritzmann, S.E., Mengel, C.E., and Fischer, C.L. "Skylab Experiment Results: Hematology Studies". *Acta Astronautica,* 2: 141-154, 1975b.

11. Konstantinova, I.V., Atropova, Ye. N., Legen'kov, V.I., and Zazhirey, V.D. "Study of Reactivity of Blood Lymphoid Cells in Crew Members of the Soyuz-6, Soyuz-7 and Soyuz-8 Space Ships Before and After Flight". *Space Biol. Med.,* 7(6): 48-55, 1973 (translation of *Kosmicheskaya Biologiya i Aviakosmicheskaya Meditsina,* 12(2): 15-19).

12. Pestov, I.D., and Geratewohl, S.J. "Weightlessness". In: *Foundations of Space Biology and Medicine* (M. Calvin and O.G. Gazenko, Eds.). Vol. 2, Book 1, NASA, Washington, D.C., 1975.

13. Taylor, F.R., and Dardano, J.R. "Human Cellular Immune Responsiveness Following Space Flight". *Aviat. Space Environ. Med.,* 54(Suppl. 1): S55-S59, 1983.

14. Talas, M., Batkai, L., Stoger, I., Nagy, K., Hiros, L., Konstantinova, I., Rykova, M., Mozgovaya, I., Guseva, O., and Kozharinov, V. "Results of Space Experiment Program "Interferon". *Acta Microbiol. Hungarica,* 30(1): 53-61, 1983.

15. Beisel, W.R., and Talbot, J.M. "Research Opportunities on Immunocompetence in Space". Life Sciences Research Office, Federation of American Societies for Experimental Biology, Bethesda, MD, December, 1985.

16. Rambaut, P.C. and Johnston, R.S. "Prolonged Weightlessness and Calcium Loss in Man". *Acta Astronautica,* 6: 1113-1122, 1979.

17. Nicogossian, A.E. and Parker, J.F., Jr. (Eds.). "Space Physiology and Medicine". *NASA SP-447,* NASA, Washington, D.C., 1982.

18. Thornton, W.E. and Rummel, J.A. "Muscular Deconditioning and its Prevention in Space Flight". In: *Biomedical Results From Skylab,* (R.S. Johnston and L.F. Dietlein, Eds.), Ch. 21, NASA SP-377, NASA, Washington, D.C., 1977.

19. Whedon, G.D., Lutwak, L., Rambaut, P.C., Whittle, M.W., Smith, M.C., Reid, J., Leach, C., Stadler, C.R., and Sanford, D.D. "Mineral and Nitrogen Metabolic Studies, Experiment M071". In: *Biomedical Results from Skylab* (R.S. Johnston and L.F. Dietlein, Eds). NASA SP-377, Washington, D.C., 1977.

20. Callahan, P.X., Schatte, C., Bowman, G., Grindeland, R.E., Funk, G.A., Leacki, W.A., and Berry, W.E. "Ames Research Center Life Sciences Payload: Overview of Results of a Spaceflight of 24 Rats and 2 Monkeys". AIAA 24th Aerospace Sciences Meeting, Reno, Nevada, January, 1986.

21. Altman, P.L. and Fisher, K.D. "Research Opportunities in Nutrition and Metabolism in Space". Life Sciences Research Office, Federation of American Societies for Experimental Biology, Bethesda, MD, February, 1986.

22. Sakahee, K., Nigam, S., Snell, P., Chue Hsu, M., and Pak, C.Y.C. "Assessment of the Pathogenetic Role of Physical Exercise in Renal Stone Formation". *J. Clin. Endocrin. and Metab.,* 65(5): 974-979, 1987.

23. Umanskiy, S.P. "Cosmonaut Equipment" (translation of "Snaryazheniya Kosmonavta," Machinostroyeniye, Moscow, pp. 1-126, 1982), *NASA TM-77192,* February, 1983.

24. Levy, M.N. and Talbot, J.M. "Research Opportunities in Cardiovascular Deconditioning". *NASA CR-3707,* 1983.

25. Nicogossian, A.E. and McCormack, P.D. "Artificial Gravity: A Countermeasure for Zero Gravity". Paper presented at the 38th Congress of the International Astronautical Federation, Brighton, England, October, 1987.

26. McCormack, P.D. "Radiation Dose Predictions for the Space Station". Paper presented at the 37th Congress of the International Astronautical Federation, Innsbruck, Austria, October, 1986.

27. Manned Mars Mission: Working Group Summary Report. *NASA M001,* Revision A, September, 1986.

28. Christensen, J.M. and Talbot, J.M. "Research Opportunities in Human Behavior and Performance". *NASA CR-3886,* 1985.

THE EFFECTS OF SPACE FLIGHT ON THE CARDIOPULMONARY SYSTEM[*]

Arnauld E. Nicogossian[†], Victoria Garshnek[‡], and F. Andrew Gaffney[†]

The human cardiopulmonary system has evolved specific mechanisms to counter the pull of gravity. In space flight, adaptation to microgravity enforces a number of alterations in cardiopulmonary physiology. The major alterations involve: 1) fluid shifts, 2) orthostatic intolerance, 3) changes in cardiac dynamics and electromechanics, and 4) changes in pulmonary function and exercise capacity. Simple but elegant experiments conducted on Space Shuttle missions have provided basic data about cardiovascular adaptation to weightlessness. Observations show that the cardiovascular system undergoes acclimation to the microgravity environment, consisting of a fairly rapid redistribution of fluids followed by a "resetting" of several controlling mechanisms. Two Shuttle flights carried ultrasound equipment (Doppler and echocardiography) for inflight determinations of central venous pressure (CVP), blood flow, cardiac dimensions, and cardiac function. Inflight echocardiography has shown a significant increase in left ventricular volume immediately after orbital insertion, which decreased as flight continued. This decrease in left ventricular volume persists for the first few days postflight, contributing to orthostatic intolerance. Measures of postflight cardiopulmonary responses to exercise have consistently revealed decreased exercise capacity, evidenced by decreases in oxygen uptake, pulse, cardiac output, and stroke volume, most of which returned to normal within 3 weeks. Submaximal exercise capacity is not adversely affected in flight, but maximal capacity has never been measured. As humans spend increasingly longer periods in space, answers to pressing physiological and clinical questions must be obtained, and effective countermeasures developed. These should evolve with further opportunities to conduct controlled studies in space.

INTRODUCTION

Gravity influences all life on Earth. It affects animal and human cardiovascular function through its hydrostatic effects on the circulation. Together with body position and responses of the peripheral circulation, gravity governs how intravascular volume is distributed and, as a result, controls heart function. Man is especially affected by gravitational changes because of his normal sitting or standing posture and

---

[*] Reprinted with permission of John Libbey Eurotext Ltd., 6, rue Blanch, F-92120 Montrouge, France, from Proceedings of the International Symposium Angiodyn 88 (Toulouse, France, Oct. 4-7, 1988).

[†] M.D., Life Sciences Division, NASA Headquarters, 600 Independence Ave., S.W., Washington, D.C. 20546.

[‡] Ph.D., The George Washington University, Washington, D.C. 20006.

because of the large body and blood volume below the heart level. The effects of gravity on the human cardiopulmonary system have long been of interest to physicians and physiologists; however, this area has received renewed emphasis with man's entry into the weightlessness of space.

In weightlessness, the body floats freely with no apparent weight . Hydrostatic pressure is eliminated, and fluids normally located in the lower regions of the body are displaced to the upper regions. This fluid shift is estimated to be as much as 1.5 to 2.0 liters in weightlessness, compared with a 500-600 ml shift when changing position on Earth (Ref. 1).

The fluid shift actually begins while the crew is supine in the spacecraft for hours in preparation for launch. In space flight, visible evidence of this fluid shift has been gleaned from photographs of the Skylab crew inflight, showing signs of periorbital puffiness and facial edema (Ref. 2). The fluid shift probably plays a major role through venous engorgement. The edema and venous engorgement do not subside even after months in space. Skylab crews also experienced nasal stuffiness and head fullness, which further support this fluid shift hypothesis.

Astronauts have typically shown inflight decrements in calf girth of up to 30%. Limb volume measured in the Skylab 4 Commander showed that lower (but not upper) limb volumes decrease early inflight and rapidly return to preflight values upon return to Earth (Ref. 2). The rate of the fluid shift appears to follow an exponential course, attaining maximum within 24 hours and reaching a plateau within 3 to 5 days (Ref. 3).

The fluid shifts result in a number of physiological readjustments. It is postulated, but not documented in flight, that the large headward shift of fluid volume rapidly induces a diuresis in response to increased right atrial pressure. In turn, this leads to a reduction in plasma volume (Ref. 4) which has been described as an actual hypovolemia, as reflected by postflight orthostatic intolerance and impaired exercise capacity (Ref. 5). A negative fluid balance with a reduction in plasma volume may also result from decreased fluid intake during the initial hours or days of a space mission. The fluid shifts trigger neurohumoral responses resulting in fluid and electrolyte changes. The size of the heart has been observed to decrease as a result of space flight (Ref. 6, 7).

Contractions of lower extremity antigravity muscles assist the return of blood to the right side of the heart. Atrophy of these muscles and changes in the ability to sustain tone can result in reduced postflight orthostatic tolerance, especially if combined with a loss in circulating blood volume. Upon return to Earth, the resulting reduction of muscle mass in the lower extremities, coupled with fluid losses and changes in antigravity muscle strength, may cause fluid pooling and a decrease in filling volume of the right side of the heart, precipitating postflight orthostatic intolerance and reduced exercise capacity. Increased translocation of intravascular fluid to the interstitial space of the lower extremity may also be a factor (Ref. 8).

SPACE FLIGHT EXPERIENCE

Cardiovascular deconditioning was first noted when orthostatic intolerance was observed in returning Mercury astronauts. Crewmembers exhibited a decrease in systolic pressure, a narrowing in pulse pressure, and a substantial increase in heart rate (Ref. 1). These symptoms were again seen in returning Gemini crewmen and were accompanied by a moderate loss of upright exercise capacity (Ref. 9, 10, 11). During flight there were no significant changes in blood pressure, ECG, or systolic time intervals. Apollo crewmen also exhibited orthostatic intolerance following flight, as well as a loss of red blood cell mass and decrements in postflight exercise capacity, including a 25% decrease in submaximal oxygen uptake (Ref. 12, 13).

Cardiovascular changes were documented for the first time inflight during Skylab missions (Ref. 14). These flights, lasting 28, 59, and 84 days, were considerably longer than previous missions. Lower body negative pressure (LBNP) tests proved to be a greater physiological stressor in space than on Earth. The greatest losses in LBNP tolerance occurred during the first three weeks of flight. Crewmen of Skylab 3 (59 days) and 4 (84 days) also exhibited elevated mean resting heart rates and increased numbers of premature ventricular contractions during exercise (Ref. 15). Although there were no decrements in bicycle exercise capacity at 50% of maximal capacity during flight, all crewmen exhibited decrements in this regard immediately following flight (Ref. 16, 17) as well as significant losses in LBNP tolerance. All crewmen wore G-suits (manually controllable cardiovascular counterpressure garments) to prevent postflight venous pooling and to reduce postflight postural hypotension.

LBNP and Physical Conditioning

Prior to the Skylab flights, it had been hypothesized that inflight LBNP would have a beneficial effect on the fitness level of astronauts, and suggestions were made to utilize this device for physical conditioning on long-duration missions. A review of Skylab LBNP data, both at rest and at 50 torr negative pressure, showed a consistent increase in both resting and stressed heart rates throughout the flights. A tendency toward stabilization of heart rate response was observed by the tenth day in Skylab, a similar finding as on STS. Most crewmembers responded with a pronounced orthostatic response postflight, with only one crewmember on the Skylab 4 mission showing a comparable response to his preflight tests. These data indicate that although LBNP might have had some favorable effects on tolerance to repeated passive cardiovascular stress as the flight progressed, only one crewmember demonstrated a beneficial postflight effect with regard to physical conditioning and orthostatic response (Ref. 8)

Space Shuttle Experience

Orthostatic intolerance became of great concern when the U.S. instituted the Space Shuttle Program in 1981. The returning crews are now subjected to the stress of gravity along the body's Z axis (head to toe) during the reentry period and are manually piloting and landing the spacecraft. In addition, postflight orthostatic intolerance could pose a hazard in the event of rapid egress from the spacecraft. This has become an even greater concern with the additional weight of the partial pressure suit and survival gear now being worn by Space Shuttle crews.

Based on bed rest studies (Ref. 18), fluid loading with a liter of normal saline prior to reexposure to gravitational stress would theoretically allow at least 40 percent of the loading volume to be maintained as increased plasma volume for up to 4 hours after ingestion. The results (Ref. 19) of this volume loading in Shuttle crewmembers showed that postflight, the countermeasure partially protected its user with a lower supine heart rate, lower standing heart rate, and the maintenance of mean blood pressure in comparison with those who used no countermeasure. However, results of postflight stand tests show that fluid loading, while beneficial, did not completely reverse orthostatic intolerance. In fact, the countermeasure appeared to be less effective after long Shuttle flights (8-10 days) than short flights (3-6 days) (Ref. 7). Factors other than hydrostatic pressure and fluid volume are probably involved and may include muscle atrophy, nervous control, resetting of baroreceptors, and passive fluid transfer to the interstitial spaces. No serious cardiovascular problems have occurred to date, but all crewmembers have been provided with G-suit protection because of the concern for decreased orthostatic tolerance postflight. Reentry heart rates have been shown to rise, attributable to the stress associated with landing and to reentry $+G_z$.

In Soviet manned space flights, extensive bicycle and treadmill exercises are used during flight as well as incremental LBNP for 15 to 20 days before reentry and ingestion of water/saline just prior to reentry. These countermeasures have not been entirely successful, as cosmonauts continue to experience significant postflight cardiovascular deconditioning (Ref. 20). Following flight, resting heart rate is slightly, but significantly, elevated in all cosmonauts.

Echocardiography

Echocardiograms were obtained pre- and postflight for the Skylab 4 astronauts during rest and LBNP stress in order to assess ventricular function. These studies demonstrated postflight decreases in stroke volume, left ventricular end-diastolic volume, and estimated left ventricular mass. The resulting data indicated that cardiac function and myocardial contractility did not deteriorate despite decreases in cardiac size and stroke volume (Ref. 21).

Additional pre- and postflight echocardiographic measurements were continued during U.S. Shuttle flights, providing additional basic data about cardiovascular adaptation to weightlessness (Ref. 7). Two routine Shuttle flights carried ultrasound equipment (Doppler and echocardiograph) for inflight determination of central venous pressure (CVP), blood flow, cardiac dimension, and cardiac function. The noninvasive (Doppler) estimates of CVP paralleled estimates obtained from subjects during Spacelab missions SL-1 and D-1, suggesting that the Doppler method can be used to monitor the time course of changes in CVP during flight. Echocardiography results showed a significant increase in the volume of the left ventricle (which propels the blood through the circulatory system) immediately after orbital insertion, with decreases as the flight progressed. Data compared with supine rest values preflight, show decreases of 16 percent in the left ventricular volume index immediately postflight, while systolic volume is changed only slightly. The net result is a decrease in stroke volume, but when coupled with increased heart rate, this results in no change in cardiac index (cardiac output normalized to body surface area).

Cardiac wall thickness is not changed and, as seen in Skylab, this implies an overall decrease of approximately 11 percent in left ventricular mass. Rapid recovery of this mass is usually seen. The precise explanation for this is unknown. These data were further enhanced by inflight echocardiographic data obtained on four crewmembers during Shuttle flight 51-D. M-mode measurements made as early as 4 hours into the mission and compared with preflight supine resting values showed that right ventricular dimension was decreased 30 percent throughout the duration of the 7-day mission and returned to preflight level immediately postflight. Whether the change in dimension represents an actual change in right ventricular volume or merely reflects changes in heart position is not known. Left ventricular diastolic volume index and stroke volume index were elevated on flight day 1 and then decreased to levels 15 percent below the preflight level. Consistent with previous data, heart rate was elevated and mean blood pressure (systolic and diastolic) remained greater than preflight levels during the mission (Ref. 22). By one week postflight, nearly all Shuttle crewmembers returned to preflight blood pressures.

The echocardiographic (left ventricular) and Doppler ultrasonic measurements (carotid flow patterns) made by French investigators during Salyut 6 (Ref. 23) indicated that left ventricular and atrial dimensions increased slowly during the early phases of flight (peaking by day 4) and then returned to baseline; carotid flow decreased during this period, then also returned to resting levels. Left ventricular end diastolic volume was decreased significantly postflight, again agreeing with earlier U.S. echocardiographic findings following Skylab flights (Ref. 21). These changes are consistent with associated postflight Skylab chest X-ray observations of decreased total heart volume (Ref. 6). It is believed that the major cause for these changes was a significant flight-related loss of intravascular volume (Ref. 24, 25, 26).

Dysrhythmias

Various levels of cardiac dysrhythmia have been noted throughout the U.S. space flight experience. During Gemini and Apollo, occasional premature ventricular contractions were seen and at least one episode of nonsustained atrial bigeminy was noted. These, however, were attributed to possible hypokalemia. During the Skylab series, all crewmen exhibited some form of rhythm disturbance, mainly rare PVCs, and, in one instance, a five-beat run on ventricular tachycardia during a lower body negative pressure testing protocol. Another crewmember had periods of wandering supraventricular pacemaker during rest and following exercise periods. These levels of dysrhythmia were greater than any shown during limited preflight ground monitoring.

In Shuttle flights, the continued prevalence of dysrhythmias was again noted. For example, during reentry, one Shuttle crewmember exhibited up to 16 PVCs per minute (Ref. 27). Sustained ventricular bigeminy was noted in an additional crewmember during extravehicular activity (however, this crewmember exhibited PVCs during preflight treadmill testing in the recovery phase of the exercise protocol). Another crewmember who showed no prior evidence of dysrhythmias exhibited sustained atrial quadrageminy during EVA. The true incidence of dysrhythmias in flight crewmembers in either 1-g or 0-g and the degree to which space flight variables, such as gravitational stress, thermal load, electrolyte changes, and catecholamine alterations, can be considered arrhythmogenic is currently unresolved.

Pulmonary Function and Exercise Capacity

Pulmonary function tests conducted postflight have generally revealed no abnormalities. However, inflight decreases in vital capacity approaching 10 percent were observed in the Skylab 3 pilot and the entire Skylab 4 crew. Results of vital capacity tests for the three Skylab 4 crewmen indicated inflight decreases, which may have been due to factors such as redistribution of body fluids, cephalad shift of the diaphragm and abdominal contents, or decrease in cabin pressure to 1/3 of sea level pressure (Ref. 28).

Postflight cardiopulmonary responses to exercise have revealed decreases in exercise capacity. Measurements obtained pre- and postflight on Apollos 7 through 11 (Ref. 29) showed significant decreases immediately postflight in workload, oxygen consumption, and systolic blood pressure. The oxygen required to perform a given amount of work (i.e. efficiency) showed no gross changes postflight. Skylab crewmen revealed similar postflight decrements in exercise capacity as evidenced by decreases in oxygen uptake, pulse, cardiac output, and stroke volume (Ref. 17). Most of these cardiovascular responses returned to normal within 3 weeks.

Studies on board Skylab and Salyut 6 demonstrated that submaximal exercise capacity is not adversely affected inflight (Ref. 17, 30, 31). Most of the Skylab crewmen exhibited increased postflight heart rates (relative to preflight baselines), but little change in heart rate during inflight exercise. Salyut cosmonauts have also shown no change in inflight performance under physical load, as reflected in measures of oxygen efficiency. Crewmembers on longer missions in both programs did not require more time for readaptation postflight. In Soviet missions lasting 96, 140, 175, and 185 days, readaptation time has not varied substantially or proportionally. In the Skylab crews, all cardiovascular parameters returned to normal within 18-21 days for the 28-day mission, within 5 days for the 59-day mission and within 4 days for the 84-day mission. Since the crew of the 84-day mission performed the most exercise inflight and the crew of the 28-day mission the least, it appears that the amount of exercise performed inflight is inversely related to the amount of time required for the cardiovascular system to readapt to Earth's gravity field. However, factors other than the amount of inflight exercise may also have contributed to these results, such as high initial levels of conditioning, loss of muscle mass, and decreased strength. Although the Skylab 3 and 4 crews started at approximately the same preflight levels of physical conditioning (as determined by oxygen consumption), a distinct improvement in VO$_2$ was noted during the last mission (Ref. 32).

FUTURE STUDIES: NEUROLOGICAL CONTROL

There is some evidence that hypovolemia alone cannot account for all of the postflight orthostatic intolerance (Ref. 33). This has led to the investigation of baroreflex regulation following head down tilt bedrest studies. Carotid baroreflex function is tested by recording the relationship between heart rate and carotid artery transmural pressure. A fiberglass and silicon neck collar connected to a motor driven bellows is used to alter the pressure of the carotid baroreceptors. The cuff pressure is typically varied from -40 to +65 mmHg. Each step is gated to the QRS of the electrocardiogram. The plot of transmural carotid pressure versus heart rate (RR interval) yields a reproducible curve characterizing baroreflex function. A recent NASA-conducted study in healthy men subjected to head-down tilt bedrest showed a decrease in the range and responsiveness of the carotid baroreflex. Comparable data will be collected before, during and after spaceflight to determine whether altered baroreflex function plays a role in postflight orthostatic intolerance as well. Additional studies of endogenous catecholamine levels and hemodynamic responses to exogenous alpha and beta adrenergic drugs will provide further information regarding the role of neural mechanisms in circulatory control immediately postflight.

CONCLUSION

Postflight orthostatic intolerance has occurred after all manned flights to date, requiring supportive care to prevent injuries and aid the process of readaptation to Earth gravity. Critical questions have arisen about how long an astronaut can continue to function efficiently and maintain acceptable physiological status inflight, and whether any of the adaptive changes that characterize cardiovascular deconditioning in microgravity may become irreversible. In order to ensure crew safety and effectiveness, more knowledge is needed on the nature and mechanisms of cardiovascular adaptation and the deconditioning that results from weightlessness; the occurrence, dimensions, and practical significance of possible regressive changes in the myocardium and other parts of the cardiovascular system; and the most effective methods of preventing or treating functional or organic deterioration of the cardiovascular system, if this does indeed occur (Ref. 34).

There is a distinct need to establish a safe and efficacious means of rehydration prior to reentry, besides ingestion of normal saline. Consideration should be given to adding glucose and other electrolytes to the normal saline in order to facilitate absorption and retention of fluids (Ref. 8). In addition, the dosage and schedule of administration should be based on carefully controlled data, not yet available. The effects of exercise, LBNP and pharmacological agents on fluid retention also requires careful study. Interventions which affect cardiovascular regulation should also be investigated in more detail, given the lack of response to saline loading alone.

In the future, humans will spend increasingly longer periods in space and will be required to perform effectively during EVA in open space or on the surface of another planetary body. As man becomes more active in Earth orbit and beyond, answers to pressing physiological and clinical questions must be obtained and effective countermeasures developed. These should evolve with opportunities to conduct controlled studies in space.

REFERENCES

1. Sandler, H. "Effects of bedrest and weightlessness on the heart". In: *Hearts and Heart-Like Organs.* G.H. Bourne (Ed.), New York: Academic Press, Vol. 2, pp. 435-524, 1980.

2. Thornton, W.E., Hoffler, G.W., and Rummel, J.A. "Anthropometric changes and fluid shifts". In: *Biomedical Results from Skylab.* R.S. Johnston and L.F. Dietlein (Eds.), *NASA SP-377,* Washington, D.C., 1977.

3. Hoffler, G.W., Bergman, S.A., and Nicogossian, A.E. "Inflight lower limb volume measurement". In: *The Apollo-Soyuz Test Project Medical Report.* A.E. Nicogossian (Ed.), *NASA SP-411,* Washington, D.C., 1977.

4. Lamb, L.E. "The influence of manned space flight on cardiovascular function". *Cardiologia,* 48: 118-133, 1966.

5. Blomqvist, C.G. and Stone, H.L. "Cardiovascular responses to gravitational stress". In: *Handbook of Physiology.* J.T. Shepherd and F.M. Abboud (Eds.), Sect. 2, The Cardiovascular System, Vol. 3. Peripheral Circulation and Organ Blood Flow. The American Physiological Society, Bethesda, MD, 1983.

6. Nicogossian, A., Hoffler, G.W., Johnson, R.L., and Gowen, R.J. "Determination of cardiac size following space missions of different durations: The second manned Skylab mission". *Aviat. Space and Environ. Med.,* 47(4): 362-365, 1976.

7. Bungo, M.W., Bagian, T.M., Bowman, M.A., and Levitan, B.M. "Results of the Life Sciences Detailed Supplementary Objectives (DSOs) Conducted Aboard the Space Shuttle from 1981 to 1986". *NASA TM-58280,* 1987.

8. Nicogossian, A., Sulzman, F., Radtke, M., and Bungo, M. "Assessment of the efficacy of medical countermeasures in space flight". Paper presented to the 37th Congress of the Int. Astronaut. Fed., Innsbruck, Austria, October 6-10, 1986.

9. Berry, C.A., Coons, D.O., Catterson, A.D., and Kelly, G.F. "Man's response to long duration flight in the Gemini spacecraft". In: *Gemini Midprogram Conference, NASA SP-121,* p. 235-263, 1966.

10. Dietlein, L.F. and Johnston, R.S. "U.S. manned space flight: the first twenty years. A biomedical status report". *Acta Astronautica,* 8(9-10): 893-906, 1981.

11. Dietlein, L.F. and Juty, W.V. "Experiment M-1: Cardiovascular conditioning". In: *Gemini Mid-Program Conference. NASA SP-121,* pp. 381-391, 1966.

12. Hoffler, C.W. and Johnson, R.L. "Apollo flight crew cardiovascular evaluation". In: *Biomedical Results of Apollo.* R.S. Johnston, L.F. Dietlein, and C.A. Berry (Eds.). *NASA SP-368,* Washington, D.C., 1975.

13. Rummel, J.A., Sawin, C.F., Michel, E.L. "Exercise Response". In: *Biomedical Results of Apollo.* R.S. Johnston, L.F. Dietlein, and C.A. Berry (Eds), *NASA SP-368,* Washington, D.C., 1975.

14. Johnson, R.L., Hoffler, G.W., Nicogossian, A.E., Bergman, S.A., Jr. and Jackson, M.M. "Lower Body Negative Pressure: Third manned Skylab mission". In: *Biomedical Results from Skylab.* R.S. Johnston and L.F. Dietlein (Eds.). *NASA SP-377,* Washington, D.C., 1977.

15. Smith, R.F., Stanton, K., Stoop, D., Brown, D., Janusz, W., and King, P. "Vectorcardiographic changes during extended space flight (M093). Observations at rest and during exercise". In: *Biomedical Results from Skylab.* R.S. Johnston and L.F. Dietlein (Eds.), *NASA SP-377,* Washington, D.C., 1977.

16. Buderer, M.C., Rummel, J.A., Michel, E.L., Mauldin, D.G., and Sawin, C.F. "Exercise cardiac output following Skylab missions. The second manned Skylab mission". *Aviat. Space and Environ. Med.* 47: 365-372, 1976.

17. Michel, E.L., Rummel, J.A., Sawin, C.G., Buderer, M.C., and Lem, J.D. "Results from Skylab medical experiment M171-Metabolic Activity". In: *Biomedical Results from Skylab.* R.S. Johnston and L.F. Dietlein (Eds.). *NASA SP-377,* Washington, D.C., 1977.

18. Johnson, P.C., Jr. "Fluid volume changes induced by space flight". *Acta Astronautica,* 6: 1335-1341, 1979.

19. Bungo, M.W., Charles, J.B., and Johnson, P.C., Jr. "Cardiovascular deconditioning during space flight and the use of saline as a countermeasure to orthostatic intolerance". *Aviat. Space and Environ. Med.,* 56(10): 985-990, 1985.

20. Kakurin, L.I. "Peculiarities in the function of human cardiorespiratory system during a six month antiorthostatic hypokinesia". *Twelfth US/USSR Joint Working Group Meeting on Space Biol. and Med.,* Washington, D.C., 9-22 Nov., pp. 1-36, 1981.

21. Henry, W.L., Epstein, S.E., Griffith, J.M., Goldstein, R.E., and Redwood, D.R. "Effect of prolonged space flight on cardiac function and dimensions". In: *Biomedical Results from Skylab.* R.S. Johnston and L.F. Dietlein (Eds.), Washington, D.C., 1977.

22. Bungo, M.W., Goldwater, D.J., Popp, R.L., and Sandler, H. "Echocardiographic evaluation of Space Shuttle crewmembers". *J. Appl. Physiol.,* 1986.

23. Pottier, J.M., Berson, M., Arbeitle, P.H., Fleury, G., Patat, F., and Guell, A. "Presentation of 'echocardiography' experiment". *Proc. 33rd Congress of the Int. Astronaut. Fed.,* Paris, France, 27 Sept.- 2 Oct., pp. 150-160, 1982.

24. Johnson, P.C., Driscoll, R.E., and LeBlanc, A.D. "Blood volume changes". In: *Biomedical Results from Skylab.* R.S. Johnston and L.F. Dietlein (Eds.). *NASA SP-377,* Washington, D.C., 1977.

25. Leach, C.S. "An overview of endocrine and metabolic changes in manned space flight". *Acta Astronautica,* 18: 977-986, 1980.

26. Leach, C.S. "Metabolic and endocrine studies". In: *A Critical Review of the US and International Research on Effects of Bedrest on Major Body Systems.* A.E. Nicogossian (Ed.), National Aeronautics and Space Administration, *NASW-3223,* pp. 81-94, Washington, D.C., 1982.

27. Bungo, M.W. and Johnson, P.C., Jr. "Cardiovascular examinations and observations of deconditioning during the Space Shuttle orbital flight test program". *Aviat. Space and Environ. Med.* 54(11): 1001-1004, 1983.

28. Sawin, C.F., Nicogossian, A.E., Rummel, J.A., and Michel, E.L. "Pulmonary function evaluation during the Skylab and Apollo-Soyuz missions". *Aviat. Space and Environ. Med.,* 47(2): 168-172, 1976.

29. Rummel, J.A., Michel, E.L., and Berry, C.A. "Physiological responses to exercise after space flight--Apollo 7 to Apollo 11". *Aerospace Medicine,* 44: 235-238, 1973.

30. Gazenko, O.G., Genin, A.M., and Yegorov, A.D. "Major medical results of the Salyut 6/Soyuz 185-day space flight". *Proceedings of the 32nd Congress of the Int. Astronaut. Fed.,* Rome, Italy, 6-12 September, 1981a.

31. Gazenko, O.G., Genin, A.M. and Yegorov, A.D. "Summary of medical investigations in the USSR manned space missions". *Acta Astronautica,* 8(9-10): 907-917, 1981b.

32. Rummel, J.A., Sawin, C.F., Michel, E.L., Buderer, M.C., and Thornton, W.E. "Exercise and long duration space flight through 84 days". *J. Am. Med. Assoc.,* 30(4): 173-187, 1975.

33. Blomqvist, C.G., Nixon, J.V., Johnson, R.L. and Mitchell, J.H. "Early cardiovascular adaptation to zero gravity simulated by head down tilt". *Acta Astronautica,* 7: 543-553, 1980.

34. Levy, M.N. and Talbot, J.M. (Eds.). "Research Opportunities in Cardiovascular Deconditioning". *NASA CR-3707,* National Aeronautics and Space Administration, 1983.

PREPARING COSMONAUTS FOR SPACE FLIGHT: SIMULATION FACILITIES OF THE SOVIET SPACE PROGRAM

Victoria Garshnek[*] and Robert Overmeyer[†]

Training on specialized simulators is one of the most important methods of preparing cosmonauts to operate spacecraft systems and perform various mission activities. The Yuri Gagarin Cosmonaut Training Center, located within Star City, northeast of Moscow, is the primary site for cosmonaut training. Trainers that simulate the space environment, develop professional skills, and combine physical sensations of space with rehearsal of operational skills are utilized. Through a comprehensive and thorough approach, the Soviets prepare their crews for future extended flights, while refining their simulation and training programs as the complexities of work in space become more clearly understood.

INTRODUCTION

Simulation facilities have played an integral role in the manned space flight effort of the Soviet Union. From the beginning, simulators provided much of the information for man-machine design factors and training requirements. They continue to be particularly important in space mission design, since there is essentially no opportunity for a graduated series of practice efforts under true operational conditions prior to mission launch.

Simulators have been employed primarily for training purposes. Since space mission crews must be trained to be highly proficient in their tasks before flight, high fidelity simulator systems are imperative for training crewmembers for specific, individual aspects of the mission (partial simulation) and for the completely integrated "dress rehearsal" (full-scale simulation) (Ref. 1). Integrated and specialized simulators are important tools for preparing cosmonauts to operate station and spacecraft systems and for practicing the entire scope of activities planned for a particular mission.

Through such training the crew learns to:

o Control spacecraft systems and equipment

o Orient the spacecraft by the Earth and Sun

o Carry out various spacecraft maneuvers

---

* Ph.D., The George Washington University, Washington, D.C., 20006.

† M.S., Martin Marietta Astronautics, P.O. Box 179, Denver, Colorado 80201.

o   Assemble and dismantle replaceable equipment

o   Detect and eliminate malfunctioning systems

o   Work as a crew during emergency situations

o   Practice interaction with each other and with ground control

o   Use flight gear

o   Practice extravehicular activity (EVA)

o   Work with onboard documentation

o   Perform activities under conditions of time deficit, insufficient information, isolation, and sensory deprivation (Ref. 2).

The basic reasons for training crews with simulators and other training devices are:

1. To ensure the correlation of operations carried out on ground-based simulators to actual space flight activities;

2. To create, during training, situations analogous to those which may arise during the space flight (both routine and emergency), to objectively evaluate the crew's response, and;

3. To identify areas of difficulty requiring further training prior to actual flight and provide the necessary practice and familiarization (Ref. 3).

FACILITIES

Star City, located approximately 30 miles northeast of Moscow, is the primary training facility for the Soviet manned space program, and is staffed by cosmonauts, doctors, training officers, and engineers. Star City has numerous buildings as well as apartments and is a self-contained entity. Located within Star City is the Yuri Gagarin Training Center. Included in the large training complex are full-size simulators and mock-ups of manned spacecraft, a water immersion tank for EVA simulations, classrooms, and other support facilities and equipment (Ref. 4).

The training devices used in the Soviet manned space program are varied in their function, purpose, effectiveness and structural design and may be divided into three general types (Ref. 5):

o   Trainers that physically prepare the cosmonaut for space flight by simulating the environments to be encountered (centrifuge to prepare for high-g landing, low pressure chamber, and aircraft in Keplerian trajectories to prepare for zero-g).

o   Trainers for developing professional skills in controlling the spacecraft and its systems (navigational, communications, approach and docking, landing, life support system simulators).

o   Trainers that combine physical sensations of the space environment with rehearsal of necessary operational skills (water tanks simulating the zero-g environment to develop EVA skills).

Physical Preparation

Keplerian Trajectory. The cosmonaut training center utilizes an IL-76 aircraft in a parabolic Keplerian trajectory, which permits the trainee to experience brief exposure to zero gravity. This particular activity is used to familiarize cosmonauts with weightlessness both for routine activities and more strenuous, potentially hazardous operations such as EVA (Ref. 6).

Low Pressure Chamber. The low pressure chamber is a stationary, hermetically sealed room where the barometric pressure can be varied. The chamber is capable of providing rapid decompression and low atmospheric pressure conditions. Space suits are worn during the training period.

Centrifuge. The centrifuge helps cosmonauts develop habits for conducting work involving high acceleration loads (such as during launch and reentry). The shoulder length of the centrifuge is 18 meters and the device is capable of producing loads of up to 30 G's. During training, centrifugal forces are increased gradually, concomitant with greater time intervals between G-force exposure. This type of training is effective for enhancing tolerance levels (cosmonauts have been exposed to transverse G-forces of up to 10-G during training). On the centrifuge shoulder is a cabin that can hold one person. The cabin is either rigidly attached or mounted in a Cardan device. The Cardan device can allow several degrees of freedom while rotating in different directions (Ref. 2). Therefore, in addition to lateral acceleration, the manned capsule can also introduce a simultaneous tumble. All information from the centrifuge is monitored during each training session.

Development of Professional Skills

Simulators. The Soyuz and Mir fixed-based simulators make it possible to sequentially rehearse and refine all stages of flight. Operational skills are perfected until they become automatic, and unforeseen or emergency situation responses are specifically developed. The final stage in preparation for a flight is a combined training session in the simulators. The flight plan proceeds in real time and lasts for several days.

o   Soyuz Trainer

The Soyuz trainer (currently Soyuz TM) simulates an entire space flight (except g-loads and weightlessness) beginning with prelaunch preparation and ending with engine cutoff and recovery procedures. Cosmonauts are trained to perform basic dynamic operations such as rendezvous, docking, orbital correction, maneuvering, and descent. The cabin corresponds completely to that of the real spacecraft, but the operation of the controls is simulated by computers. The adjacent computer and control room is used to monitor the crew's performance and creates simulated emergencies to which the crews can respond.

o   Docking Simulator

The docking simulator is an exact duplication of the actual device used to dock the Soyuz spacecraft to the space station. Special lights simulate sun light and illuminate the model exactly as it would be in the actual space flight condition.

o   Assembly Simulator

The assembly simulator is used to train cosmonauts for assembly work in space. Using the multipurpose equipment which it contains, cosmonauts are expected to assemble various structures that will eventually be brought to the space station by the Soyuz TM spacecraft, visiting crews, or unmanned cargo ships.

o   Tool Simulator

Exercises with onboard tools are performed on a simulator. During this training, cosmonauts are familiarized with the variety of tools and where they are kept, training in assembly-disassembly and repair-restoration-replacement work. They learn how to approach the units to attach instruments, acquire skills in using the tool, and study the technical servicing instructions.

o   Electromechanical Starry Sky Simulator

Leading scientists in the USSR participate in training cosmonauts in the areas of astrophysics and space navigation. A special planetarium at the Gagarin Cosmonaut Training Center, built with the assistance of the German Democratic Republic, precisely recreates some 900 constellations and stars of the Celestial Sphere. Movements of the moon and planets are simulated by a Cardan device.

Space Station Mock-Ups. Using mock-ups of orbital stations, and even the stations themselves (before they are placed in orbit), cosmonauts are able to rehearse and perfect the procedures and skills needed for unloading cargo spacecraft, refuelling station thrusters, performing experiments, and carrying out reactivation work while on board. Cabins of the mock-up trainers are equipped with actual life support systems, communications, and medical and scientific equipment. The tasks at this stage of cosmonaut preparation are the development and clarification of flight assignments, obtaining initial baseline physiological data utilizing actual onboard systems, and performing work for long periods of time.

Combined Simulation: Physical Preparation/Skill Building

To prepare cosmonauts for EVA, great emphasis is placed on simulating weightlessness during training sessions. Under these conditions cosmonauts practice operations involving cargo handling, egress into space, transfer between spacecraft, installation of solar panels, along with assembly, dismantling, and repair work.

Hydrolaboratory. The Gagarin Cosmonaut Training Center is equipped with a special water immersion facility called the Hydrolaboratory, which is fitted with a telemetric measuring complex as well as film and video equipment (Ref. 3). The large immersion tank (hydropool) fully contains a specially prepared mock-up of the current orbital station and additional spacecraft in docked configuration.

Wearing special pressure suits, the cosmonauts spend long periods of training in simulated weightlessness under water. Lead weights are placed into the suit's pockets to give its wearer zero buoyancy. The hydrolaboratory provides an effective simulation of space, since it produces high emotional loads, requires an artificial atmosphere, produces a condition of "weightlessness" and necessitates the use of special equipment.

SIMULATOR CONTROL: THE COMPUTER COMPLEX

Analog and digital computers with large storage and high response capability are used to control various simulators and certain training devices. These computers are able to control the trainers and simulators, monitor crew performance, provide simulated malfunctions to test crew alertness and training; and store, process, and output the information. In the past, space simulators were independently functioning facilities, each with its own computer, visual simulation system and control panel. As a result of the growing number of crews involved with simulation training, the construction of simulators as independently functioning units became outdated, both economically and technically. This necessitated transition to a new basis of integrated training facilities, making use of comprehensive systems (computer, data bank and others), with the aim of allowing simultaneous use of many simulators, life-size mock-ups, and other devices (Ref. 3).

FUTURE/CONCLUSIONS

The broad application of modern computer and data bank technology lays the foundation for increasingly thorough and qualitative solutions to the problems of training crews to perform tasks of greater complexity and sophistication. Envisioned for the future is the modelling of a wider range of emergencies to expand the scope and level of actions to be taken in emergency situations, greater control of the level of training, and further automating the planning and control of cosmonaut training. Much attention is being placed on enhancing the methods and procedures necessary to accomplish important scientific research, which increases every year as a result of the growing duration of space flights and the rising numbers of experiments carried on board (Ref. 3).

Sustained, high-quality performance of crews in space is necessary for their safety and for the successful completion of mission tasks. It is evident that the Soviets are utilizing a comprehensive and thorough approach to prepare their crews for future, extended flights, while continuously refining their simulation and training programs as the complexities of work in the space environment become more clearly understood.

REFERENCES

1. Connors, M.M., Harrison, A.A., and Akins, F.R. "Living Aloft: Human Requirements for Extended Space Flight". *NASA SP-483,* NASA, Washington, D.C., 1985

2. Bluth, B.J., and Helppie, M. *Soviet Space Stations as Analogs,* 2nd Edition. NASA Headquarters, Washington, D.C., August, 1986. P. III-102-119.

3. Shatalov, V. "The Training of Cosmonauts", In: *History of the USSR: New Research:* 5. Nauka Press, Moscow, 1986.

4. Committee on Science and Technology House of Representatives. 99th Congress, 1st Session, Serial 1. Visit to Sweden and the Soviet Union. Report prepared by the Subcommittee on Space Science and Applications. U.S. Govt. Printing Office, Washington, D.C., 1985.

5. Gurovskiy, F.P., Kosmolinskiy, F.P., and Mel'nikov, L.N. "Designing the Living and Working Conditions of Cosmonauts". *NASA TM-76497,* NASA, Washington, D.C., May, 1981.

6. Committee on Commerce, Science, and Transportation: U.S. Senate Part 2., *Soviet Space Programs: 1976-1980* (Supplement 1983). U.S. Govt. Printing Office, Washington, D.C., 1984.

LONG-DURATION SOVIET MANNED SPACE FLIGHT: THE DEVELOPMENT AND IMPLEMENTATION OF POSTFLIGHT RECOVERY MEASURES

Victoria Garshnek[*]

Since the mid-1970s, Soviet scientists have utilized and improved upon a structured postflight recovery program consisting of rehabilitative measures to help cosmonauts readapt to Earth's gravity and recertify them for flight status as soon as possible. Generally, the following recovery measures are taken: therapeutic measures to restore orthostatic stability and tolerance to light exercise; application and gradual expansion of physical exercises; massage of muscles, sport games and outdoor sports to restore coordination; sauna, and psychoemotional activity. The effectiveness of these measures is judged on the basis of subjective evaluations, heart rate, and blood pressure in the course of the procedures and scheduled clinical examinations. Recovery measures are conducted initially at the landing site and Star City, and then at a mountain health resort. Observations of cosmonauts after long-duration space missions indicate that the effectiveness of rehabilitative measures increases with proper scheduling of the daily regimen, optimum alternation of exercise and rest, combined with positive psychoemotional factors. Over the years the Soviets have also observed that optimal use of inflight physiological countermeasures seems to improve the ease and speed of postflight recovery. Regardless of the actual effectiveness of inflight countermeasures, the gradual process of postflight rehabilitation will undoubtedly continue. Since inflight countermeasures used thus far have not been totally effective against weightlessness, further improvements in the recovery program and rehabilitative treatments may assume greater importance as manned space flights continue to be incrementally extended and should a weightless flight to Mars (requiring 2-3 years) be pursued in the future.

INTRODUCTION: HISTORICAL PERSPECTIVE

With the establishment of reliable space stations and safe crew transport vehicles by 1975, the Soviets have possessed the necessary resources in space to investigate human physiological and psychological capabilities and limitations. With further space station sophistication, consistent incremental extensions in flight duration were possible. This trend has progressed into the present day (Table 1).

Previous space flights have indicated that cosmonauts develop various physiological changes that create some difficulties for them upon return to Earth's gravity. The difficulties arise from changes in motor function and fluid-electrolyte balance, deconditioning of the cardiovascular system for exercise and orthostatic

* Ph.D., The George Washington University, Science Communication Studies, Washington, D.C. 20006.

tolerance, decreased mineralization of bone tissue, anemia, muscle atrophy, and pain in the muscles and ligaments. Similar changes have also been induced by antiorthostatic hypokinesia and immersion (Ref. 1). The observed data indicated that use of preventive measures inflight (countermeasures) and appropriate rehabilitative methods postflight, might provide an added advantage or margin of safety in readapting to Earth's gravity after long-duration missions.

Table 1

PROGRESSIVE INCREASES IN SOVIET LONG-DURATION FLIGHT TIME

Year	Station	Long-duration Flight Range (Days)
1975	Salyut 4	29 - 63
1976	Salyut 5	49
1977-81	Salyut 6	75 - 185
1982-86	Salyut 7	65 - 237
1986- Present	Mir	125 - 326

The search for appropriate methods for rehabilitating cosmonauts after extended flights began in the 1970s. The first combined rehabilitative and therapeutic measures for the postflight period were developed in ground-based studies using the model of 49- and 182-day antiorthostatic hypokinesia as well as from general clinical experience (Ref. 2, 3, 4). The 49-day study showed that the efficacy of rehabilitative measures increased with proper scheduling of the daily regimen, optimum alternation of exercise and rest, combined with positive psychoemotional factors in the form of special autotraining sessions, psychotherapy, and appropriate musical accompaniment to exercises.

The principles of rehabilitative measures developed after the 49-day antiorthostatic hypokinesia study served as the foundation for developing systems of combined rehabilitation and therapy for the 182-day study. After 182 days of antiorthostatic hypokinesia, particularly in the group of test subjects who did not use preventive measures (countermeasures such as exercise, etc.), the recovery period lasted up to 2 months. Normalization of the cardiorespiratory and neuromuscular states occurred 7-10 days earlier in groups where preventive measures were used during the hypokinetic period (Ref. 5).

The preventive and rehabilitative methods that were developed during these studies served as the basis for rehabilitative therapy following 140- and 175-day space flights (Salyut 6, 1978-79). The general scheme established during this time is still, with certain modifications and improvements, followed today.

GENERAL STRUCTURE OF THE RECOVERY PROGRAM

From observations of recovery both postflight and after antiorthostatic hypokinesia, Soviet scientists have concluded that physiological readaptation after long-duration flight or hypokinesia generally follows certain stages. For example, during the first few days postflight, changes are distinct, with symptoms manifesting during rest and under negligible orthostatic or physical loads. This progresses (by approximately 1 week) to a state where physiological disturbances develop with orthostatic and physical loads of average intensity. About 1 month postflight, restoration of function is seen during load tests. Finally,after approximately 1.5 months, return to a normal or near-normal functional state and efficiency is achieved.

These general physiological stages have served as a guide for timing various rehabilitative activities in the development of a postflight recovery program for cosmonauts. The therapeutic recovery measures are also individualized and are constantly adjusted on the basis of speed of recovery, pulse rate, arterial pressure, and other postflight medical data, as well as subjective reports from the cosmonauts themselves.

Postflight rehabilitative therapy is conducted in two stages:

- o Stage I: Begins at the landing site and continues at Star City (2 weeks)

- o Stage II: Conducted at a Caucas Mountain health resort (approximately one month).

Stage I

During stage I, the cosmonaut's physical condition is gradually and carefully restored to the point of orthostatic tolerance, capacity for light exercise, and relief of muscle pain. During this first phase, the chief means of rehabilitative therapy consists of motor activity, therapeutic massage of muscles, graded walking, hydrotherapy and thermotherapy, and autogenic conditioning, as well as diet, vitamins, and drug therapy (Ref. 5).

0-2 Days. The anti-g suit is worn during reentry and transport to Star City and may be worn up to 4 days postflight. On the day of landing, therapy is limited to relaxation massage of the muscles combined with autogenic training to remove fatigue and emotional tension, and heat-water treatment to relieve emotional stress, muscle pain, and improve circulation. Therapy also includes dietary measures such as multivitamin supplements and drug therapy. During the first few days, morning toning exercises are performed including small and medium muscle exercises and breathing exercises (no more than a 50% increase in pulse rate) (Ref. 5). Walking in anti-g suits is limited to indoors with subsequent rest. Massage is conducted 2-3 times a day after physical loads or functional tests and is differentiated as relaxing or toning depending on the state of muscle tone. Relaxation exercises and heat treatments are carried out in the evening. During the first few days postflight, cosmonauts may be excited, emotionally uplifted, gesticulating, making abrupt movements, wanting to get up, etc. Physicians and therapists frequently find it necessary to restrain cosmonauts' physical activity because of their desire to force the amount and intensity of motor activity (Ref. 6). Cosmonauts are cautioned against performing abrupt movements or walking sharply and are encouraged to do purely supporting movements.

The first postflight walk is a measured walk (i.e., walking with assistance, medically supervised, and controlled for heart rate in an anti-g suit). This initial walk can take place during the first or second day postflight (Ref. 7,8). For example, the day after his 326-day flight, Yuri Romanenko walked his first 100 steps, supported by his wife and crew physician (Ref. 6). During the initial stage, cosmonauts generally have noted cardiovascular lability and some soreness in the back and leg muscles (Ref. 9).

3-10 Days. After 3 days postflight, limited physical workouts begin. Water calisthenics in a swimming pool (27°C) and exercises for average and large muscle groups are included, and walking at variable speeds in combination with breathing exercises are begun. Each day the volume and intensity of exercise is expanded. Duration and intensity of walks (unaided) increase, reaching 10-14 km by postflight days 8-10 (Ref. 5,9).

10-14 Days. Toward the end of the first stage (about postflight day 10) the number and duration of water and heat treatments (sauna) are expanded. Massage during this period includes rubbing and kneading of the back and lower legs. Physical activities are increased to include running, jogging (with walking pauses), bicycling, volleyball, and table tennis. Heat treatments are combined with contrasting temperature treatments to aid vascular and muscle tone. The cosmonauts may even be able to take some personal time off on the weekends or holidays to go fishing or pursue personal endeavors instead of the rehabilitative therapy.

At the end of Stage I, cosmonauts are generally feeling better and their readaptation progress can be considered as satisfactory. By this time the feeling of gravity becomes more usual (Ref. 10). However, cosmonauts may still tire easily and reduced orthostatic stability, decreased tone of the antigravity muscles, and slight uncoordination may still persist (Ref. 9).

At the end of the 2-week stage I period, the cosmonauts are transported to another time zone (Caucas mountain resort) for continuation of therapy (Ref. 5, 11).

Stage II

The recovery therapy begun in stage I is continued during stage II in a resort setting. The beneficial climate, which includes a large number of sunny days even in autumn and winter, moderately high altitude, the variety of outdoor running trails, and the wide range of bath and physical therapy facilites are believed to be instrumental in enhancing the recovery process after long-term space flights (Ref. 11). All of the available facilites are utilized: swimming pool, athletic complexes and equipment, tonic and relaxed muscle massage, walking trails, sea bathing, whirlpool baths, etc.

During the initial days at the resort facility, therapy is conducted at a reduced pace and loading in order to acclimate the cosmonauts to the higher elevation (about

3,300 feet or 1,000 meters) and time change. During this stage significant individual differences in readaptation are usually seen.

After acclimatization to resort conditions, physical training is performed with the use of a "three-peaked" physiological curve of physical load (Ref. 5). Cosmonauts also have more free time during this stage, and greater individualization of rehabilitative measures is possible. Balenological therapy (mineral baths) is also added to the rehabilitative routine.

POSTFLIGHT MEDICAL TESTS

A variety of postflight medical examinations and biochemical tests are conducted during the recovery period (Ref. 12, 13). These examinations include the following:

o   Clinical examination

o   Investigation of the cardiorespiratory system and hemodynamics at rest and during provocative tests

o   Evaluation of motor activity, motor control, and vestibular function

o   Investigation of fluid-electrolyte metabolism and renal function

o   Investigations of bone density

o   Anthropometric measurements

o   Biochemical investigations (blood enzymes, blood lipids, carbohydrates, nitrogen, vitamins, and hormones)

o   Hematological investigations

o   Immunological investigations

o   Microbiological investigations

o   Subjective questionnaires.

The postflight recovery period is an important source of biomedical information. Not only do the results help to improve future recovery program structure, but they also provide some insight into the progression and success of physiological reversibility (in some systems), which is vital for incremental increases in flight duration to continue.

CONCLUSION

Long-duration human space flight is one of the most ambitious physiological experiments of our time. Since 1977, man has tolerated long-term weightlessness for periods raging from 96 days up to 1 year. Already the 17 individuals who have flown 96 days or more have demonstrated that man can indeed tolerate space flight conditions of long duration up to 1 year and return to Earth with the ability to recover and return to work.

The Soviets have indicated that by the end of these recovery measures, cosmonaut condition improves considerably (Ref. 7, 9, 11). However, serious questions remain to be answered if a voyage to Mars (accomplished in a weightless state) is to be given serious consideration. Is there a critical duration of weightless exposure beyond which irreversible physiological changes take place? Is there a limit to the duration spent in weightlessness beyond which the 1-g recovery period would be extremely difficult to endure? How cautious and careful must postflight rehabilitative procedures be after a 2-3 year period of weightlessness and reduced gravity?

Quite possibly, the question of concern may not be whether humans can survive a weightless trip to Mars and back, but rather, will the space travelers be able to effectively exit their spacecraft and work efficiently on the planet's surface under the influence of 1/3-g? Indeed, with these questions in mind, the postflight recovery period becomes much more interesting and important to observe as further extensions in flight duration continue and missions to the planets are seriously contemplated.

REFERENCES

1. Krupina, T.N. and Tizul, A.Ya., *Soviet Med.* (in Russian), No. 7, pp 30-34, 1978.

2. Kabanov, M.M., *Vestn. Amn. SSSR* (in Russian), No. 4, pp. 52-58, 1978.

3. Danilov, Yu. Ye., Gazenko, O.G., and Fedorov, B.M. et al., *Vopr. Kurortol.* (in Russian), No. 1, pp. 39-44, 1976.

4. Sorokina, Ye. I., Kanevich, N.A. and Daninov, B.I., *Sov. Med.* (in Russian), No. 1, pp. 73-77, 1978.

5. Krupina, T.N., Beregovkin, A.V., Bogolyubov, V.M., Fedorov, B.M., Yegorov, A.D., Tizul, A.Ya., Bogomolov, V.V., Kalinichenko, V.V., Ragulin, A.P., and Stepin, V.a. "Combined Rehabilitation and Therapeutic Measures in Space Medicine". *Sovetskaya Meditsina* (in Russian) No. 12 pp. 3-8, Dec. 1981.

6. Moscow Television Service (in Russian), 1530 GMT 30 Dec. 1987, from the "Vremya" newscast.

7. Yegorov, A. D. "Results of Medical Studies During Long-Term Manned Flights on the Orbital Salyut-6 and Soyuz Complex". *NASA TM-76014.* National Aeronautics and Space Administration, Washington, D.C., 20546, November, 1979.

8. *Moscow Literaturnaya Gazeta* (in Russian), p. 2, February 3, 1988.

9. Gazenko, O.G., and Yegorov, A.D. "175-day space flight: some results of medical investigations". *Vestnik,* USSR Academy of Sciences, No. 9, 1980.

10. Moscow Television Service (in Russian), 1530 GMT 8 January, 1988, from the "Vremya" newscast.

11. Gazenko, O.G. (Ed.) "Rehabilitative measures after long-term space flights in a health resort in the city of Kislovodsk". *Space Biology and Aerospace Medicine: Abstracts of Papers Delivered at the Eighth All-Union Conference,* Kaluga, 25-27 June 1986. (In Russian) Moscow: Nauka, 1986.

12. Vorobyov, E., Gazenko, O.G., Genin, A.M., and Egorov, A.D. "Medical Results of Salyut-6 Manned Space Flight". *Aviat. Space Environ. Med.* Supp. 1, 54(12): S31-S40, 1983.

13. Gurovskiy, N.N. (Ed.) *Results of Medical Research Carried Out Aboard "Salyut-6" - "Soyuz" Orbital Complex.* (In Russian) Moscow, Nauka Press, 1986.

APPENDICIES

SPACE PHOENIX PROJECT[*]

OVERVIEW

The SPACE PHOENIX Program is a joint effort of a nonprofit university consortium and its commercial project manager to develop a program for the safeguard-
ing and subsequent utilization of the U.S. Shuttle fleet's expended external fuel tanks
for scientific and commercial purposes, with the goal of seeing near-Earth space
opened up to as many people, organizations and activities as rapidly as possible, and
at the lowest possible cost.

These organizations are the University Corporation for Atmospheric Research
(UCAR), the UCAR Foundation (both of which are nonprofit organizations) and
the External Tanks Corporation (ETCO; a for-profit organization). The UCAR
Foundation is the majority stockholder in ETCO.

UCAR, a 28 year-old group of 57 universities and research institutions, has requested title for the right to use all the discarded external tanks (ETs) of the U.S.
Shuttle fleet. The economy of scale shall permit UCAR, through its project manager
ETCO, to safeguard these assets as a National Trust and make them readily available
to the scientific and industrial community for scientific and commercial purposes
using private funds. Space flight engineers have concluded that this undertaking is
technically and operationally possible, thereby creating valuable assets from these
used and previously discarded ETs.

The SPACE PHOENIX Program is similar in many respects to the university
land grant program, where land was awarded to universities in the previous century
in the expectation that they would contribute to the development of the nation. In
this age, the Shuttle fleet's large ETs can be thought of as analogous to parcels of raw
land in space. The grant by NASA would also contribute to the economic development of the Nation.

The SPACE PHOENIX Program premises that UCAR will obtain title for the
right to use ETs in space in the form of a fiscally neutral "space grant" from the
Federal Government. Such a grant would permit ETCO to arrange private financing
to accomplish the modification, outfitting and management of the ET resources. The
UCAR Foundation's share of the net income and asset value developed from such

---

[*] This document is reprinted with permission of UCAR and ETCO. Any questions or comments should be directed to
Peter Riva, ETCO, Marketing & Public Relations, 116 East 95th Street, New York, New York 10128. The document
includes the revised draft for space policy. This is version SPPOL05PR, and incorporates revision by Dr. R. Ware, B.
Marks and P. Riva, March 1, 1988.

uses will provide a long-term endowment that will be employed to benefit the university scientific community.

Anticipated innovative collaborations between government, universities and commercial organizations; the challenging financing, engineering, operating and management issues; the creation of a National Trust of ETs; the potential for the creation of wealth in orbit; the important implications for civil space development in space science, transportation and commerce facilities -- all call for a bold and imaginative national commitment to the SPACE PHOENIX Program.

The University Corporation for Atmospheric Research (UCAR) is a private, nonprofit corporation organized as a consortium of 57 institutions which acts as a national scientific research nucleus (Nb. 1). Founded in 1959, it has grown steadily from the original 14 charter universities to its present membership. The growth of its membership testifies to the increased importance of atmospheric and related studies in the nation's higher education and research system.

The dynamic relationships among the Earth's atmospheric layers, its oceans and the solar-interplanitary environment, cause UCAR's working definition of "the atmosphere" to include regions bounded by the oceans' floor, extending to the sun and out toward the edge of the planetary system. Atmospheric scientists have long utilized remote-sensing spacecraft to observe phenomena in this vast realm and UCAR's scientific involvement in space-related activities has a lengthy history. UCAR participated in the utilization of Skylab, the world's first manned orbiting observatory, and has shared major responsibility in the design of satellites, instruments, experiments and in-space repair facilities. UCAR's growing interest in obtaining and utilizing orbiting scientific facilities within atmospheric space is a logical and consistent development of its charter, which includes the development of extensive and complex research tools and making such tools available to scientists in national and international communities.

UCAR also leads research projects on behalf of the overall atmospheric sciences community and coordinates such efforts with its 57 member institutions and other academic and research institutions throughout the world that are expert in atmospheric, computer and related sciences. UCAR has a particular capability in bringing government and university groups together to achieve common scientific goals, carrying out research efforts at various times for the National Science Foundation (which provides its principal support), NASA, the Department of the Navy, the Federal Aviation Administration, the National Oceanic and Atmospheric Administration, the Department of the Air Force, the Environmental Protection Agency and other government and non-government entities.

In August 1987, UCAR convened a symposium to consider the use in space of the expended External Tanks of the U.S. Shuttle fleet for scientific purposes (Nb. 2).

THE UCAR FOUNDATION

The UCAR Foundation was established to enhance and conserve the value of the "commercial spinoffs" from ongoing scientific research programs, to provide administrative flexibility in dealings with the private sector and to seek opportunities for the creation of wealth to be used to advance scientific research (Nb. 3).

The U.S. Government has recognized that knowledge-intensive high-technology industries have long-term implications for international competitiveness, thereby affirming the economic benefits of scientific research. Universities and research institutions such as UCAR, which play a central role in creating knowledge, presently receive more than $8 billion annually from the taxpayer in support of basic, civilian, scientific research. This research frequently yields significant practical discoveries and technologies, benefiting the public and causing valuable stimulation of the economy.

To promote this kind of activity and accelerate technology transfers between academic and industrial sectors, the Congress passed Public Law 96-517 in 1980. This legislation permits academic institutions to own title to discoveries and inventions developed with government support in their laboratories, thus encouraging them to share in the economic values generated by their research efforts. This expanding pool of intellectual property has highlighted the potential benefits to be derived from imaginative university-industry collaborations. This trend has led to mutually beneficial long-term strategic partnerships between members of the academic and corporate worlds, sometimes involving hybrid and novel institutional forms, thus strengthening support for scientific activity.

UCAR, in common with many other research organizations, examined the challenges involved in owning intellectual properties (and other assets such as corporate gifts), as well as the need for dealing with the private sector in business terms. The Board Of Trustees of UCAR decided in 1986 to establish the UCAR Foundation to act as fiduciary and to direct and manage certain intellectual properties and other unique assets on behalf of UCAR.

In addition to the SPACE PHOENIX Program, the UCAR Foundation is engaged in assisting UCAR with technology transfer and commercialization issues deriving from programs such as "Airport Of The Future", Doppler radar technology (which promises early warning of sudden atmospheric downdrafts - microbursts - near airports) and the commercial development by Mesa Archival Systems, Inc. of mass data file transfer software for supercomputers.

THE EXTERNAL TANKS CORPORATION

The External Tanks Corporation (ETCO) was created as a Delaware (for-profit) corporation to manage the private financing, development, storage and operation of Shuttle fleet expended fuel tanks for scientific and commercial uses in space. The UCAR Foundation holds a majority of the shares of ETCO, the remainder being held by directors and investors (Nb. 4).

SHUTTLE EXTERNAL TANKS

The Space Shuttle's External Tank (ET) is designed to carry the liquid fuels that power the main engines of the Orbiter and to serve as a "strongback" on which the the Orbiter and the pair of solid fuel boosters are mounted (see Figure 1). Currently, just before insertion into orbit, the Orbiter crew jettisons the ET, which reenters the dense lower regions of the atmosphere, burns and breaks into pieces which fall into the ocean. During a Shuttle launch, the reusable solid boosters exhaust their fuel after about 2 minutes and then separate for recovery, while the ET continues to fuel the main engines for another 6.5 minutes until orbital velocity is approached and the ET is separated (Nb. 5). To date, 24 ETs have been jettisoned in this controlled and safe fashion.

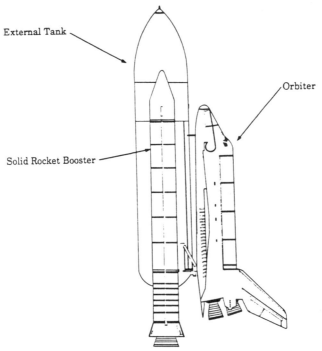

External Tank

Orbiter

Solid Rocket Booster

Figure 1   Space Transportation System

ETs consist of 27 metric tons (60,000 pounds) of strengthened aluminum, 1980 cubic meters (70,000 cubic feet) of separate pressurized hydrogen and oxygen vessels, and an intertank section (see Figure 2) with a non-pressurized volume of 141.5 cubic meters (5,000 cubic feet). The Shuttle Cargo Bay can carry 20 metric tons with a volume of 285 cubic meters (10,000 cubic feet). An ET has a 8.4 meter (27.6 feet) diameter and a 46.5 meter (153 feet) length. It is roughly the size of a Boeing 747 body.

The concept of using ETs as environments for work and scientific study is reminiscent of Skylab, which was fashioned from the upper stage fuel tank of a Saturn 5 rocket. In 1976, space experts within NASA suggested it was feasible to put ETs into near-Earth orbits where their potential value could be realized without (significant) payload loss or increased launch cost (Nb. 6). Other experts in the aerospace industry and academia agree that orbiting laboratory-habitat facilities could be created economically from expended ETs by outfitting them with life-support, station-keeping, communications and power elements (Nb.7). Auxiliary equipment needed to modify and use ETs could be carried in the Orbiter Cargo Bay or within the non-pressurized ET intertank structure or in an "aft cargo carrier" behind the ET or by expendable launch vehicles.

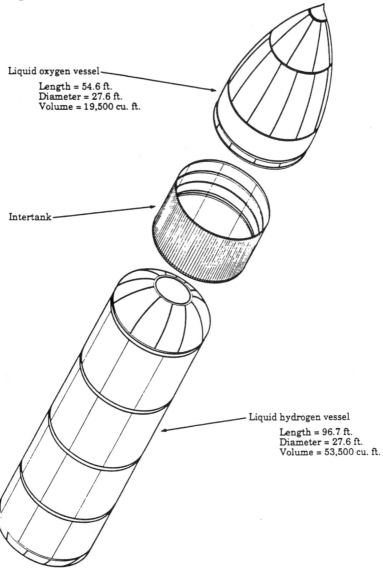

Liquid oxygen vessel
  Length = 54.6 ft.
  Diameter = 27.6 ft.
  Volume = 19,500 cu. ft.

Intertank

Liquid hydrogen vessel
  Length = 96.7 ft.
  Diameter = 27.6 ft.
  Volume = 53,500 cu. ft.

Figure 2 External Tank Structure

The manufacturing cost of a single ET is about $30 million and post-Challenger estimates of the cost to launch payloads into low-Earth orbit, based on a fully operational Shuttle fleet, are up to $13,200 per kilo ($6,000 per pound). Therefore, an ET retained in orbit and not destroyed represents roughly a third of a billion dollars of launch cost as a national asset. The 27 metric tons of strengthened aluminum and other material from which ETs are constructed, the 1980 cubic meters of pressurized volume, the 4 to 7 metric tons of residual fuels and the large mass, strength and structure of the ETs are all valuable space resources. Due to their mass and strength, ETs are particularly well suited to tether applications, including momentum transfer between orbiting bodies and the creation of artificial gravity.

OFFICIAL VIEW

In 1982 the U.S. Congress requested its Office Of Technology Assessment (OTA) to carry out a study on civilian space stations (Nb. 8). It became obvious to OTA staff that ETs might be transformed into valuable space assets. Following an open workshop convened by NASA it was concluded that ETs could be used in orbit in a variety of ways and that:

"... an ET should be put in space at the first reasonable opportunity." (Nb. 9).

In 1986 NASA's Marshall Space Flight Center demonstrated their evolving seriousness toward seeing ETs used in space by awarding a contract to Martin Marietta Aerospace Corporation to study scientific and engineering questions related to turning an ET into a valuable scientific resource, initially, its transformation into a very large unmanned orbiting Gamma-Ray Imaging Telescope (Nb. 10). Astronauts would enter an ET through the existing 91 centimeter (36 inch) aft manhole port and then assemble telescope components within the empty hydrogen vessel. The vessel would be resealed and pressurized to provide the required experimental environment.

The National Commission on Space, a Presidentially-appointed panel of space specialists, referred to the use of ETs in its report as follows (Nb. 11):

"... there is a potentially valuable artificial resource that is now going to waste: the Shuttle's external tanks. At present, with each successful flight of a Shuttle, an empty tank with a mass greater than the full payload of the Shuttle itself, is brought to 99 percent of orbital speed and then discarded to burn up in the atmosphere. The Shuttle fleet's flight schedule suggests that over a 10 year period about 10,000 tons of that tankage will be brought almost to orbit and then discarded. At standard Shuttle rates, it would cost about $35 billion to lift that mass to orbit."

In the U.S. Congress, the House of Representatives' Committee on Science, Space and Technology referred specifically to the use of ETs in orbit and to NASA's verification of the feasibility of such use in a section entitled "Utilization of Orbiting Shuttle External Tanks" in its final report accompanying the NASA Authorization Act of 1988 (Nb. 12):

"The committee notes that the Space Shuttle External Tank (ET) is a potentially valuable resource that should be considered for possible space development. Qualified academic research groups could be awarded ET resources for space-based research much like the land grant concept of the past. Using orbital ETs, universities working cooperatively with industry might be able to increase scientific research opportunities, expand our Nation's space infrastructure and broaden the spectrum of private space enterprise.

In response to the Committee's request in House Authorization 99-829, NASA has delivered to the Committee a report specifying the technical, operational, cost and safety requirements for ET orbit insertion. The NASA report "External Tank Utilization on Orbit" states:

"The engineering and operating problems involved with this objective are basically within the current state-of-the-art of Shuttle operations, support system and technology." The report also specifies the impact on Shuttle payload, propellant requirements for station keeping, requirement for accessibility for orbiting ETs, probability of space debris or micrometeoroid damage and NASA's estimate of the cost of ET modifications and operations. The Committee appreciates the delivery of this detailed report in response to the Committee's specific request.

The Committee is pleased to be informed of progress achieved by university groups and NASA in the past year toward realizing the potential value of ET resources: (1) The University Corporation for Atmospheric Research (UCAR), a 25 year old group of 57 universities and research institutions, is leading the "Space Phoenix" program to obtain orbiting ETs and develop them for scientific and commercial purposes using non-government funds; (2) NASA has created a high level committee to work with UCAR on the Space Phoenix program; (3) UCAR and the Government are making good progress towards an agreement concerning the transfer of one or more ETs to UCAR; (4) NASA is supporting studies of a Gamma Ray Imaging Telescope (GRIT) which would be installed in an orbiting ET; (5) Zero Gravity simulations of GRIT telescope assembly procedures are being conducted at the Marshall Space Flight Center; (6) A symposium of space scientists has been convened by university groups to consider space experiments that can be conducted in and from space using ETs."

On February 11, 1988, the White House released "The President's Space Policy and Commercial Space Initiative to Begin the Next Century" which states on pp.2, item II:

"The President is announcing a fifteen point commercial space initiative to seize the opportunities for a vigorous U.S. commercial presence in Earth orbit and beyond -- in research and manufacturing. This initiative has three goals:

Promoting a strong U.S. commercial presence in space;

Assuring a highway to space; and

Building a solid technology and talent base."

In the 15 point list that follows, the release states on pp.3, Point 4:

"External Tanks: The Administration is making available for five years the expended external tanks of the Shuttle fleet at no cost to all feasible U.S. commercial and nonprofit endeavors, for uses such as research, storage, or manufacturing in space."

THE SPACE PHOENIX PROGRAM

UCAR has increased its focus on space related experimental research and in the autumn of 1984, UCAR staff and some of the individuals who are now ETCO Directors began to contemplate the early use of ETs for in-space work and research facilities. Drawing on their considerable space science experience and appreciation for the general potential of in-space ETs (and the actions required to realize this potential), they concluded that orbiting ETs could and should be converted into valuable scientific facilities for atmospheric and space science research. In 1985 a task force was convened by UCAR to explore the matter in greater detail. The conceptual details of rendezvous and modification of ETs to create scientific support platforms

141

in various low Earth orbits have continued to be examined by UCAR. As a result of these investigations, the "Space Phoenix" task force developed firm confidence in the future value of utilization of in-space ETs by science and commerce for the ultimate benefit of the national scientific and university community.

The UCAR Foundation, through ETCO as its appointed project managing corporation, has begun to obtain private sector financial support to store, develop and use ETs as orbiting "research parks" for scientific and commercial purposes. In this way, universities could obtain (for commercial development) discarded government property in a manner analogous to a "land grant", potentially alleviating the substantial national backlog of demand for scientific and commercial research facilities in near-Earth orbit and opening up space for a large number and variety of public and private activities.

The UCAR - UCAR Foundation - ETCO program was named SPACE PHOENIX to signify future ETs as "rising" from the charred remains that, until, now, have marked the end of their journey to the threshold of space. The major objective of the Program is to endeavor to "save" all the ETs, whether or not of immediate scientific or commercial use and park them in a high altitude (multiple decade) orbit in a "Nest" to safeguard their potential value for future generations. ETs stored in this manner will form a "National Trust".

Another important element of the Program is to see that measures are taken (by defining the uses to which each facility could be put and utilizing already developed technology wherever possible) to produce relatively "Spartan" facilities. By keeping costs as low as possible in this manner, the Program would encourage widespread use of the ETs by national and international scientific communities.

A formal agreement, between UCAR, the UCAR Foundation and ETCO, gave ETCO the responsibility for financing, studying the scientific, legal and economic feasibility of using ETs in space for research and commercial purposes, and developing technical, engineering, business and operating plans for the enterprise. UCAR in turn agreed to accept grants of ETs after jettison and to convey to ETCO, through the UCAR Foundation, sole rights to manage ET resources in space.

In October, 1986, a committee was formed by NASA at its headquarters to analyze and explore with UCAR and ETCO the technical and programmatic implications of the SPACE PHOENIX Program. Chaired by NASA's General Manager, the other committee members are NASA's Comptroller, General Counsel and Heads of the Commercial Programs and Advanced Planning Offices. Following the first meeting of SPACE PHOENIX representatives with the NASA committee, a Memorandum Of Understanding (MOU) was signed by NASA and UCAR. The MOU (see Appendix E) states:

"NASA and UCAR believe it is in the Nation's interest to see the concept of employing external tanks for additional useful purposes explored. Therefore, NASA and UCAR agree to cooperate with each other and exert every reasonable effort to explore the concept and provided the concept proves to have merit, take appropriate further steps to bring it to fruition".

From a policy standpoint, this is completely consistent with Public Law 98-361 (modifying the 1958 Space Act) which states that NASA should

"... seek and encourage, to the maximum extent possible, the fullest commercial use of space."

In 1986, the Business-Higher Education Forum reinforced the need for multi-institutional commitment in the development of commercial space utilization and stated in their report (Nb. 13):

"All levels of government management with roles in space activity should clearly understand, and be encouraged to support, commercial development objectives, with a clear view toward nurturing a culture more supportive of entrepreneurial efforts."

THE NEED FOR SCIENTIFIC FACILITIES IN SPACE

Prior to recent launch failures, there was a five-year backlog for the launching of scientific, military and commercial space payloads. Since then, two-thirds of the planned flights of Spacelab, a system of pressurized modules and open pallets that are deployed in the Orbiter's Cargo Bay, have been cancelled or substantially postponed. The Ulysses solar-polar mission, the Galileo Jupiter mission and the Mars observer mission have been postponed and most Shuttle based space experiments are yet to be rescheduled. There is now the probability that national security related priorities will further preempt available transportation capacity, placing a further strain on the serious backlog situation.

The need for laboratory, commercial and science facilities in space is rapidly growing. In September 1986, the U.S. pledged its support to a 70 nation Earth observation program, sponsored by the International Council of Scientific Unions (ICSU), to study disturbing changes in Earth's atmosphere (for example the "Greenhouse Effect"). With critical reliance on orbital monitoring, the International Geosphere-Biosphere Program was pledged support from NASA, the National Oceanic and Atmospheric Administration, the National Science Foundation, other federal agencies and the National Academy of Sciences. The transcending importance of understanding changes in our global climate and the size of the commitment required, led the Chairman of the U.S. delegation to ICSU to call the pledged effort the "largest scientific program ever mounted."

Authorities and organizations, such as the Space Science Board of the National Academy of Sciences, involved in the creation of policy for scientific space endeavors, recognize that the scientific community requires facilities and laboratories in orbit that can support a broad range of research. This need, widely echoed throughout the scientific world, is borne out by the variety of efforts, national and international, to create permanently orbiting cost-effective habitats and uninhabited platforms for scientific investigation (Nb. 14). ETs are efficient resources for conversion to facilities of this kind and would permit private sector activities to compliment and enhance the key role planned for the U.S. Space Station (Nb. 15).

Available, cost effective, pressurized environments are of significant importance to man's exploration of space. Human ingenuity and flexibility in the deployment, assembly, operation, maintenance and repair of scientific facilities define the need for

143

and the design of habitable pressurized environments as work spaces in near-Earth orbits. There are also a great many important and valuable scientific programs which do not require people to remain in orbit. These pressurized or shielded containers have unique values, as in microgravity experiments, life science experiments or for radiation imaging telescopes. On the other hand, for many scientific efforts, crew-time is the resource which limits the rate of progress or success. A recent study by NASA, which analyzed prior and future space missions, concluded that, on the grounds of cost effectiveness alone, there was no substitute for humans in space (Nb. 16).

In either configuration, with or without resident professionals, the backlog of demand for permanent in-space science-related infrastructure is considerable. In short, an orbiting "research park" promises to be in the position of leasing occupancy to a prestigious international list of scientific and commercial tenants who need access to high volume, low cost, facilities for relatively long periods of time.

Support for space-related research and commercial activities pervades many sectors of scientific and financial planning at federal agencies and research institutions and business corporations. Funding of research and development in the U.S. exceeds $100 billion annually. Approximately half that amount is spent by private sector corporations, with the balance funded primarily by the federal government. Significantly, demand for cost-effective orbiting laboratory habitats is found in a very broad section of research, commercial and development programs. Placing aside the important agendas in applied space science, development and engineering, the current basic research backlog covers a number of fields, facilities and activities (see Appendix F). The sums now budgeted by NASA, the European Space Agency (ESA) and Canada for space-related scientific research approach a total of some $2 billion per year. These sums will grow, probably significantly, by the turn of the century. Expenditures for a wide range of business activities including communications, insurance, health care, clothing, food, legal services and engineering will become increasingly important.

The ongoing efforts of a growing number of aerospace firms and foreign countries to develop commercial space exploration capabilities promise to augment the total international launch capacity available to the world's scientific community. Those who choose to explore and conduct approved scientific work in space, will need pressurized containers and specialized scientific facilities and services, whether financed by research institutions or by private companies. ETs could become basic resources for all of these science-related activities and thereby serve important cultural and economic roles on a large scale.

THE UCAR SYMPOSIUM ON SCIENTIFIC USE OF EXTERNAL TANKS

A symposium on "The Scientific Use of Orbiting Shuttle External Tanks", supported by NASA, Martin Marietta Aerospace Corporation and the Universities Research Association, was convened by UCAR on August 3 and 4, 1987 in Boulder, Colorado (see Nb. 2). Invited space scientists exchanged and developed ideas on potential scientific experiments that would utilize ETs in the areas of astronomy and astrophysics, life sciences, material sciences and remote sensing. In addition to suggestions for specific experimental use of ET facilities in these areas, it was widely recommended that the 141 cubic meters (5,000 cubic feet) of non-pressurized volume in the ET Intertank section be used to carry experiments as soon as possible. Initially, the Intertank area could be utilized during sub-orbital flights, thereby reducing the backlog of low altitude scientific payloads and also serving as a first step toward wider use of ET resources.

OBTAINING RIGHTS TO USE EXTERNAL TANKS

The SPACE PHOENIX Program premises that UCAR shall obtain the right of use for the Shuttle fleet's ETs and then, through ETCO, its program manager, arrange for independent financing, modification, outfitting, operation, maintenance and management. Assignment of ownership rights for such novel assets requires a policy decision by the Government and the recipient of such rights must be an entity that can be expected to serve the national interest. The rationale of the SPACE PHOENIX Program is that, by having a vested interest in developing ET in-space scientific and commercial facilities, members of the 57 institution UCAR consortium will apply their ingenuity to the challenge of creatively salvaging and recycling, for a wide variety of third party users, space "scrap" having unique chemical, physical and structural properties. As ET resources become progressively developed and widely used in the scientific, commercial and government sectors, activities of this kind would generate rewarding returns.

Such efforts would necessarily involve a large and long-term collaborative partnership among the academic community, the business sector, banking and financial institutions, and agencies of the Federal Government. The creation of intersectoral relationships of this kind are now constantly being evoked by the nation's policy makers. Evolving the specific novel institutional and organizational forms that would be necessary, is believed to be no less challenging a task than realizing the overall civil in-space ambitions of the U.S. during the coming century.

As the logical and suitable choice to receive such a "space grant", UCAR's accomplishments are significant. It has a 27 year history as manager of the National Center for Atmospheric Research, one of the most prestigious and productive scientific laboratories in the world. UCAR exists as a joint effort of 57 leading research institutions and is broadly representative of U.S. academic research interests. Additionally, UCAR has been historically involved with a large number of scientific activities that must be conducted from space. While the Congress has the authority to grant such rights for ETs (and shall play the decisive role in such a determination), current Public Law also vests similar authority in the NASA Administrator (Nb. 17):

> "[to award]... any items of a capital nature... which may be required... for the performance of research and development contracts... to nonprofit organizations whose primary purpose is the conduct of scientific research... [if] the Administrator determines that the national program of aeronautical and space activities will be best served... [by doing so]."

A parallel may be drawn to the Morrill Act of 1862 in which raw land was awarded to universities as "land grants". As with the case of a "space grant" of ETs, the cost to the government is minimal. Neither the 1862 or the present grant involves budgetary appropriations, and both include the expectation that universities would develop such resources to realize economic gains to support education activities and the broadest national interest. This has proven true in the experience of the "land grant" history and the same is expected for a future "space grant". Legislation proposing federal financial support for universities involved in space research has been passed by the Congress (Nb. 18). Given the current and projected federal deficit and consequent budget criteria, a "space grant" of ET physical assets (currently discarded) presents itself as an alternative, and fiscally neutral, initiative.

The Congress has previously granted space related rights with much the same progressive and constructive outcome: in 1964 the transfer of rights to the Comsat program was made as a fiscally neutral grant of "communication rights". This bold and far reaching Congressional action has caused the creation of a multi-billion dollar space communications industry which, in turn, has assured American world dominance in this vital arena, increasing technology and creating tens of thousands of jobs.

The formidable demand for extra-terrestrial scientific facilities reflects a backlog of primary research, whose dimensions run across the years to the training and education of whole categories of scientific personnel and to the design of experiments that require significant lead times. The nation's articulated science agenda in space has lead to a "baseline configuration" for the present U.S. Space Station Program which provides the country with its essential infrastructure in the global competition to develop space, an event of great historical importance.

Through approximately the end of this century, the Space Station program contemplates a basic nucleus of five flexible integrated pressurized modules with a total core volume, U.S. and foreign, of some 850 cubic meters (30,000 cubic feet). To a very large extent, the future public civil activities of the U.S. in space will rest upon this centerpiece facility. Yet, its ability to support in-space scientific inquiry is limited. While it is difficult to quantify the difference between the amount of research that scientists are seriously interested in seeing carried out in space and the capacity of the Space Station to support such research, it appears that the difference is substantial (Nb. 19). Since NASA presently estimates that it will require some twenty Shuttle missions during 1994 and 1996 to assemble the core of the Space Station it is challenging to contemplate that over 40 times the quantity of raw pressurized ET tank volume (36,620 cubic meters) would be discarded under current Shuttle deployment methodology. UCAR's privately financed retrofitting of ETs in orbit would significantly compliment and enhance the strategic utility (and long range value) of the centerpiece U.S. Space Station.

A joint public-private approach in support of the extraordinary human enterprise of developing space should be in the best interest of all parties. The economic context must evolve from today's near exclusive dependence on Government appropriations towards a shared program wherein private investment supports the expansion of private space exploitation and where business requirements for return-on-investment begin to emphasize large scale more efficient activities and to constrain costs. This methodology will bring about an altogether more economically sound and dynamic exploitation of space.

CONCLUSIONS

Unanimous agreement on the potential utility and economic value of ETs cannot, in itself, provide for the safe placement in orbit or conversion of expended ETs into orbiting facilities. In addition, this event is unlikely to occur if dependant on appropriations of Federal funds because of understandable competing demands in the civil space budget. The SPACE PHOENIX Program, as planned by the UCAR - UCAR Foundation - ETCO partnership, is as different from NASA "cutting edge" technology and Government infrastructure as the covered wagon-train was to the Lewis and Clarke expeditions; both fulfill vital and irreplaceable functions in the development of America.

Once again, the time has come when the Government's efforts to trail-blaze, develop and exploit space need to be augmented through a determined and innovative intersectoral program. SPACE PHOENIX brings the ingenuity of UCAR, the UCAR Foundation, and ETCO, together with the Federal Government and the private sector, to bear on the challenge of using ETs, safely, and without burden to the taxpayer. SPACE PHOENIX is an exciting pioneering step in the development of the space frontier.

REFERENCES

1. UCAR is a private, nonprofit corporation organized under the laws of the state of Colorado, and has the following 57 member institutions: University of Alaska, University of Arizona, California Institute of Technology, University of California at Davis, University of California at Irvine, University of California at Los Angeles, University of Chicago, Colorado State University, University of Colorado, Cornell University, University of Denver, Drexel University, Florida State University, Georgia Institute of Technology, Harvard University, University of Hawaii, University of Illinois at Urbana-Champaign, Iowa State University, Johns Hopkins University, University of Maryland, Massachusetts Institute of Technology, McGill University, University of Miami, University of Michigan, University of Minnesota, University of Missouri, Naval Postgraduate School, University of Nebraska at Lincoln, University of Nevada, New Mexico Institute of Technology, State University of New York at Albany, New York University, North Carolina State University, Ohio State University, University of Oklahoma, Oregon State University, Pennsylvania State University, Princeton University, Purdue University, University of Rhode Island, Rice University, Saint Louis University, Scripps Institution of Oceanography at the University of California at San Diego, Stanford University, Texas A&M University, University of Texas, University of Toronto, Utah State University, University of Utah, University of Virginia, University of Washington, Washington State University, University of Wisconsin at Madison, University of Wisconsin at Milwaukee, Woods Hole Oceanographic Institution, University of Wyoming, Yale University. Members of the UCAR Board Of Trustees are listed in Appendix A.

2. "Report on the Scientific Use of Orbiting Shuttle External Tanks Symposium," Center for Space and Geosciences Policy, University of Colorado, October, 1987.

3. The Officers and Directors of the UCAR Foundation are listed in Appendix B.

4. The Officers and Directors of ETCO are listed in Appendix C. Advisors to ETCO are listed in Appendix D.

5. While the destruction of Challenger and the loss of its crew will lead to significant technical changes in the Space Transportation System, the causes of the January 1986 disaster did not involve the external tank, and no changes are expected to be made to it. A comprehensive investigation of the event by the Presidential Commission exonerated the tank as a cause of the calamity: "The Commission reviewed the External Tank's construction records, acceptance testing, pre-launch and flight data, and recovered hardware and found nothing relating to the External Tank that caused or contributed to the cause of the accident." (Report of the Presidential Commission on the Space Shuttle Challenger Accident, June 6, 1986, Washington, D.C., p. 41).

6. "External Tank Utilizations for Early Space Construction Base", NASA Marshall Space Flight Center, December, 1976.

7. The report, "Space Shuttle External Tank Applications" includes 95 references on the use of expended ETs in space. Space Studies Institute, Princeton, NJ, December, 1985.

8. "Civilian Space Stations and the US Future in Space", Office of Technology Assessment, Government Printing Office, November, 1984.

9. "Report by the External Tank Working Group," California Space Institute, University of California at San Diego, March, 1983.

10. Koch, D., "External Tank Gamma Ray Imaging Telescope Study". Final Report, Contract A71128 (for Martin Marietta Corp.), Smithsonian Astrophysical Observatory, Cambridge, Massachusetts, 1987.

11. "Pioneering the Space Frontier," p. 84, Bantam Books, May, 1986, p.84.

12. "National Aeronautics and Space Administration Authorization Act, 1988", Report 100-204, July 7, 1987, p. 22. The NASA Authorization Act, 1987, included similar recommendations in a section entitled "External Tanks as Space Assets", Report 99-829, September 16, 1986, pp. 32-33.

13. "Space: America's New Competitive Frontier", Business - Higher Education Forum, Washington, D.C., August, 1986. This report was issued by a task force under the co-chairmanship of the President of the California Institute of Technology, and the Chairman and CEO of Rockwell International Corporation. It was recommended for wide distribution by the Forum membership of 42 university presidents and 41 corporate CEOs.

14. See, for example, "Research in Space: Prelude to Commercialization", G.A. Hazelrigg, Jr., and M.E. Hymowicz, prepared at the National Science Foundation for presentation at the 37th Congress of the International Astronautical Federation (IAF), October, 1986.

15. Although the pressurized volume of a single ET is twice the total of that planned for the U.S. Space Station, the use of ET volume planned by the SPACE PHOENIX Program is more limited in scope. The facilities would play quite different, yet complementary roles. Whereas Space Station will see many sophisticated, necessarily expensive, "cutting edge" technologies developed and used for the first time, recycled single purpose ETs will draw upon technology that is already developed and has been space qualified in such programs as Skylab, Spacelab and Shuttle. ET facilities could relate to Space Station in the way that warehouses relate to high-tech research facilities on earth.

16. The Human Race in Space, NASA -- CR 171223, September, 1984.

17. National Aeronautics and Space Administration Authorization Act of 1986, Public Law 99-170.

18. "A Bill to Establish a National Space Grant College Program", Senate Bill S.2098, February 25, 1986.

19. Crew size will be confined to some half dozen persons owing to the size limitations of the Space Station. The "overhead" demanded by such functions as service, diagnostics, repair, logistics, maintenance, assembly, communications, arrivals and departures, exercise, rest, recreation, eating and sleeping, will further constrain the productive time and number of personnel available for scientific research.

SELECTED PHOTOGRAPHS OF SPACE MEDICINE
RELATED ACTIVITIES

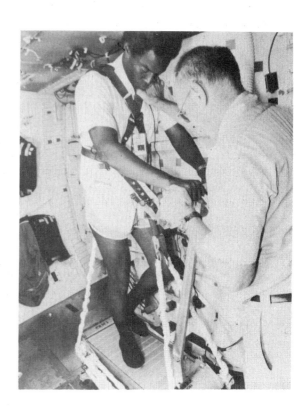

Fig. 1 Dr. William E. Thornton, right, and Guion S. Bluford, both mission specialists for STS-8, demonstrate an on-orbit experiment in the Johnson Space Center's one-g trainer. The treadmill device was designed by Dr. Thornton and has been used on previous Shuttle flights (NASA Photo Nos. 83-HC-519, 83-H-606, S-83-37627).

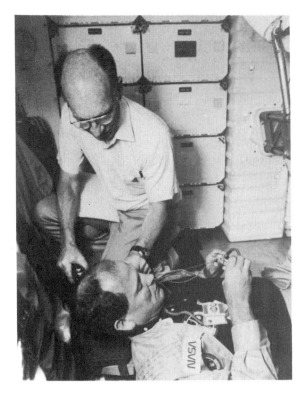

Fig. 2 Dr. William E. Thornton (in street clothing) conducts a medical test on Dr. Norman E. Thagard as the two astronauts prepare for mission specialist duties on STS-7 (June 1983) and STS-8 (Aug.-Sept. 1983). This training session included a demonstration of the evoked potentials experiment. Dr. Thornton is principal investigator on a number of past and future Space Shuttle medical experiments as well as serving "in the field" with the third Challenger mission's battery of tests and experiments. The two doctors are pictured in the Johnson Space Center's one-g trainer (NASA Photo Nos. 83-HC-520, 83-H-607, S-83-34144).

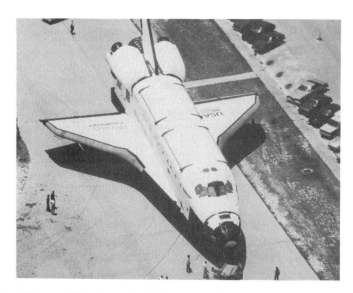

Fig. 3 Challenger's roll from the Orbiter Processing Facility to the Vehicle Assembly Building is underway as preparations continue towards launch of the eighth Space Shuttle, Kennedy Space Center, Florida (NASA Photo Nos. 83-HC-540, 83-H-633, 108-KSC-83PC-533).

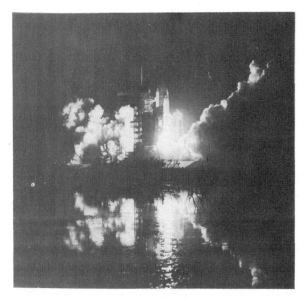

Fig. 4 The Space Shuttle lights up the predawn sky as it lifts away from Complex 39's Pad A to begin the STS-8 mission with the first nighttime launch of the Shuttle era. Challenger's blastoff came 17 minutes late at 2:32 a.m. after mission managers prolonged the final built-in hold until weather conditions became acceptable. The evening's earlier rain storm failed to dampen enthusiasm for the spectacular sight of the Shuttle's departure on a planned six-day flight. The mission will also end in darkness with the Shuttle gliding to a nighttime touchdown on the concrete runway at Edwards AFB, California (NASA Photo Nos. 83-HC-566, 83-H-663).

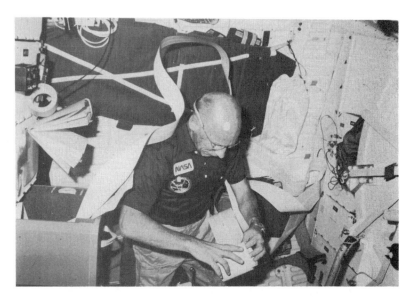

Fig. 5 Astronaut William E. Thornton, a very busy mission specialist conducting a great deal of biomedical experimentation on STS-8 mission, checks a prolific roll of data in the mid-deck of the Earth-orbiting Space Shuttle Challenger. The electrode on Dr. Thornton's forehead indicates that his four crewmates were not his only test subjects during th extensive tests on this six-day flight (NASA Photo Nos. 83-HC-572, 83-H-670, S08-14-0378).

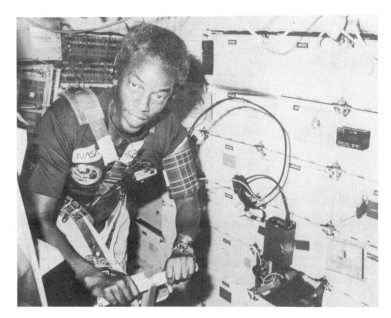

Fig. 6 Astronaut Guion S. Bluford, STS-8 mission specialist, assists Dr. William E. Thornton (out of frame) with a medical test that requires use of the treadmill exercising device designed for space flight by the STS-8 medical doctor (NASA Photo Nos. 83-HC-580, 83-H-678, S08-13-0361).

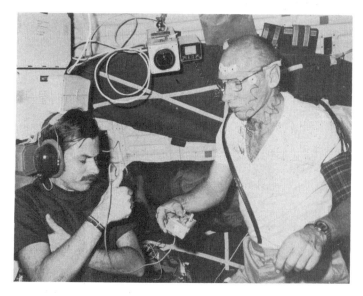

Fig. 7 Astronaut William E. Thornton (right) conducts an audiometry test on Astronaut Dale A. Gardner in the mid-deck of the Earth-orbiting Space Shuttle Challenger STS-8. Both men were mission specialists for the reusable spacecraft's second five-person crew. This frame was shot with a 35mm camera (NASA Photo Nos. 83-HC-583, 83-H-681, S08-18-0468).

152

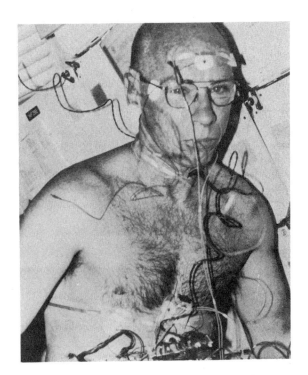

Fig. 8 Dr. Thornton undergoes self-conducted medical testing onboard the Challenger STS-8. He has electrodes placed around his eyes to monitor movement of the eyes and some non-related narrow strip tape electrodes on his forehead, around the neck and chest as part of the ambulatory monitoring system, this portion being impedance cardiography (NASA Photo Nos. 83-HC-600, 83-H-700, SL08-09-0229).

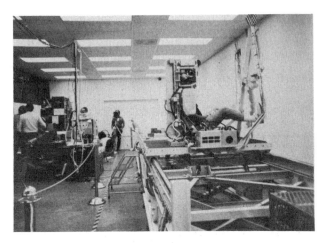

Fig. 9 In the Baseline Data Collection Facility (BDCF), located at NASA's Ames-Dryden Facility, STS-9 Spacelab 1 Mission Specialist Robert A.R. Parker conducts an experiment on a computer-driven linear acceleration laboratory sled. The BDCF sled, mounted on two 30-foot steel rails with teflon bearings, can accelerate to 0.6 g's and has built-in redundant safety mechanisms. Six experiments, part of the Spacelab 1 investigations, are conducted using the BDCF sled. The various experiments are designed to help scientists learn more about the human body's gravity-sensitive organs in the inner ear. The BDCF is a laboratory equipped to record pre-flight and post-flight data for life science investigations examining the body's adaptations and responses to stresses associated with increasing time spent in space and its residual effects. Pre-flight data is recorded in the BDCF at 90,60,30 and 11-day intervals prior to launch. This photo depicts testing at an F-(minus) 30 data gathering. The BDCF is located at Ames-Dryden, a part of NASA's Ames Research Center, so post-flight data recording can begin as soon as possible following landing (NASA Photo Nos. 83-HC-706, 83-H-832, ECN-26764).

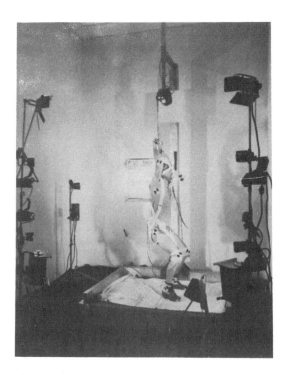

Fig. 10 In the Baseline Data Collection Facility (BDCF) located at NASA's Ames-Dryden Facility, STS-9 Spacelab 1 Mission Specialist Owen K. Garriott is "dropped" as part of an Experiment that investigates the vestibulo-spinal reflexes associated with balance organ responses and the relationship of space motion sickness to the investigation results. During the experiment, the crewman is "dropped" unexpectedly from the drop station a distance of 6-8 inches while a mild electric shock is applied to the tibial nerve in his calf muscle. When the shock is applied, the tibial nerve conducts signals throughout the nerve cell pool in the spine and back down to the postural muscles in the calf of the leg. This reflex is measured, as are vertical eye movements, acceleration and the duration of the fall; high speed motion pictures are taken. This experiment is also done in space during the Spacelab 1 mission (NASA Photo Nos. 83-HC-707, 83-H-833, ECN-26750).

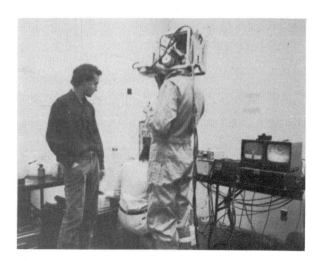

Fig. 11 In the Baseline Data Collection Facility (BDCF), located at NASA's Ames-Dryden Facility, experimenters prepare STS-9 Spacelab 1 Mission Specialist Robert A.R. Parker for an experiment, 1ES201, that studies eye movements, postural adjustments, and illusions of attitude and motion evoked by eye movement stimuli to assess visual-inner ear interaction. Parker is standing on a circular platform which can tilt, creating motion for postural adjustments. Over his head is a helmet-like device which has a TV camera over the left eye and visual display over the right eye showing various eye movement stimuli giving the illusion of motion. Eye movements are recorded and TV monitors, shown on the right, enable the experimenter to observe the eye movements (NASA Photo Nos. 83-HC-708, 83-H-834, ECN-26735).

Fig. 12 Researchers assist STS-9 Spacelab 1 Mission Specialist Byron K. Lichtenberg in preparation for the Dark Lab and Tilt Table (1ES201) experiment in the Baseline Data Collection Facility (BDCF) at NASA's Ames-Dryden Facility. In darkness, constrained in a roll-axis tilting, rigid harness, the crewman faces a luminous line mounted on a black rotatable disk. While his eyes are closed, the line is rotated. He then opens his eyes and signals when he thinks the line is back to a vertical position. Researchers expect continued perceptual improvement as the vestibular (balance organ) system begins to readapt to a one-g environment. Eye movements including ocular torsion or rotation are recorded for this experiment (NASA Photo Nos. 83-HC-716, 83-H-841, ENC-26760).

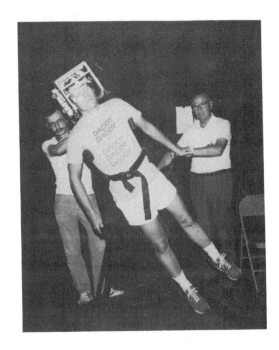

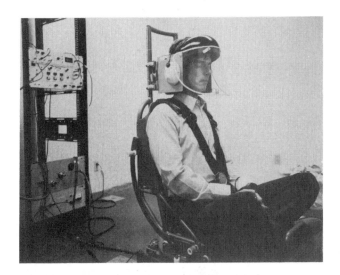

Fig. 13 STS-9 (Columbia) Spacelab 1 Payload Specialist Ulf Merbold participates in the Benson Linear Threshold Detection Device (BLTDD) experiment (1ES201) used to measure the crewman's ability to detect low threshold level acceleration. Located in the Baseline Data Collection Facility (BDCF) at NASA's Ames-Dryden Facility, the BLTDD consists of a lightweight movable seat that runs on an air bearing surface. The crewman's eyes and ears are covered to help prevent tactile sensations of movement and the experiment is performed in a low light-level room. The tests are conducted in several body positions (NASA Photo Nos. 83-HC-716, 83-H-842, ENC-26742).

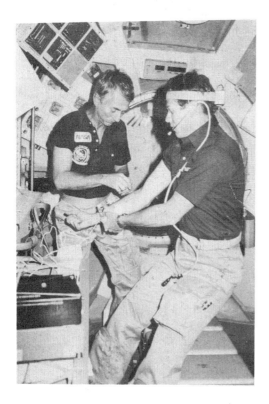

Fig. 14 Owen Garriott draws blood from
Byron K. Lichtenberg (STS-9 Columbia)
for later testing on Earth (NASA Photo
Nos. 83-HC-736, 83-H-870, S09-50-143).

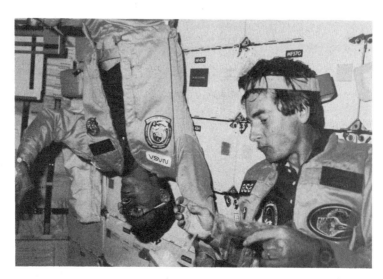

Fig. 15 John Young and Ulf Merbold during a meal in the mid-deck of Columbia (STS-9). Merbold's "head
band" is part of a test to monitor the payload specialists during their waking hours throughout the mission
(NASA Photo Nos. 83-HC-737, 83-H-871, S09-30-075).

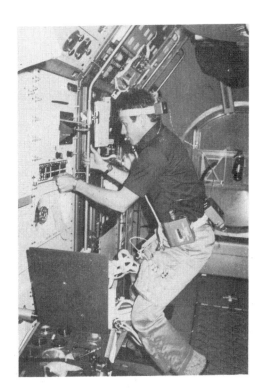

Fig. 16 Byron K. Lichtenberg at the materials Science double rack facility (Experiment 300), a project of ESA. More than 30 different experiments for investigators from nine European nations were performed here during the STS-9 flight (NASA Photo Nos. 83-HC-738, 83-H-872, S09-30-068).

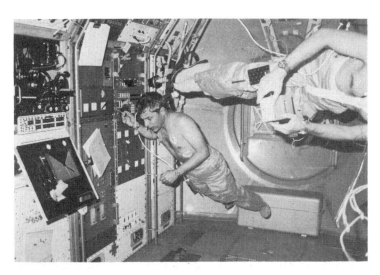

Fig. 17 With a great deal of "ground" to cover in a few days' time, versatility became an important trait onboard Spacelab, as depicted in this photograph. Astronaut Robert A.R. Parker, left, floating in the microgravity environment, participates in a biomedical test along with the unidentified crewmember at the right. But it appears recent attention has been devoted to the materials science double rack facility (left edge), as the protective shield for the fluid physics module has been removed (NASA Photo Nos. 83-HC-745, 83-H-879, S09-07-0527).

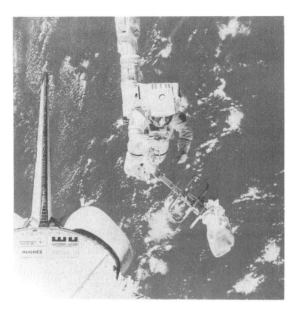

Fig. 18 Astronaut Bruce McCandless II, on February 7, 1984 (Flight 41-B) used the combination of the Remote Manipulator System (RMS) arm and the Mobile Foot Restraint (MFR) to experiment with a "cherry-picker" concept (NASA Photo Nos. 84-HC-94, 84-H-91, 584-27037).

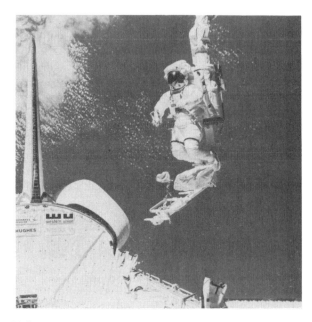

Fig. 19 Astronaut Bruce McCandless II, on February 7, 1984 (Flight 41-B) uses the combination of the Remote Manipulator System (RMS) arm and the Mobile Foot Restraint (MFR) to experiment with a "cherry-picker" concept (NASA Photo Nos. 84-HC-97, 84-H-94, 584-27040).

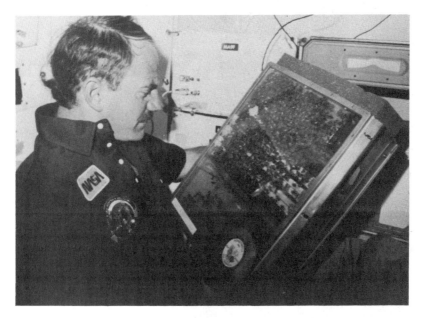

Fig. 20 Astronaut James D. van Hoften, 41-C Mission Specialist, holds an aluminum box, full of honeybees. The experiment in Earth orbit is duplicated with another colony of the young honeycomb builders on Earth. Dan Poskevich submitted the experiment to NASA as part of the Shuttle student involvement program (NASA Photo Nos. 84-H-161, 84-HC-173, S18-5-188).

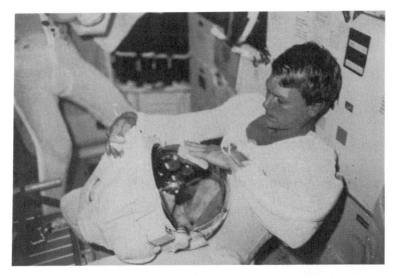

Fig. 21 Astronaut George D. Nelson, 41-C Mission Specialist, wipes off his helmet visor in the mid-deck of the Earth orbiting Space Shuttle Challenger. Astronaut James D. van Hoften, Mission Specialist, who joined Dr. Nelson for two Extra-Vehicular Activities (EVA) on this seven-day flight, is seen in the background. Both crewmembers are wearing the liquid cooled undergarments for the Extravehicular Mobility Unit (EMU) (NASA Photo Nos. 84-H-163, 84-HC-175, S13-12-0423).

Fig. 22 A magnificent Earth limb photograph of a sunset as seen from orbit off the coast of Rio de Janeiro, Brazil, shows thunderheads overshooting into the stratosphere more than 10 miles (16 kilometers) high and flatting at the tropopause. The violet hues of the limb continue to a height near the base of the ionosphere at an altitude of almost 50 miles (80 kilometers). The photograph was shown by crewmembers during the STS-41D postflight press conference held on September 12, 1984 (NASA Photo Nos. 84-H-514, 84-HC-458, S14-3214).

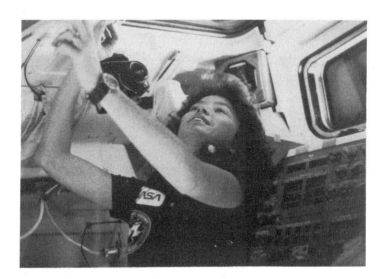

Fig. 23 Anna L. Fisher, is pictured in this 35mm frame near the aft flight deck of Discovery, where she remained very busy on November 12 & 14, 1984 while fellow crewmembers worked to retrieve two stranded communications satellites (NASA Photo Nos. 84-H-646, 84-HC-573, S19-20-004).

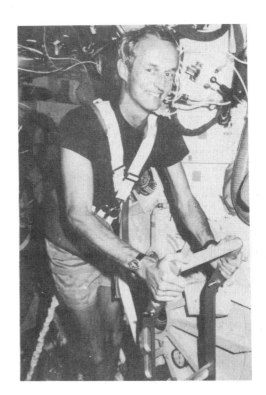

Fig. 24 Donald E. Williams, pilot, works out on the treadmill exercising device in Discovery's mid-deck (NASA Photo Nos. 85-H-139, 85-HC-114, 51D-05-017).

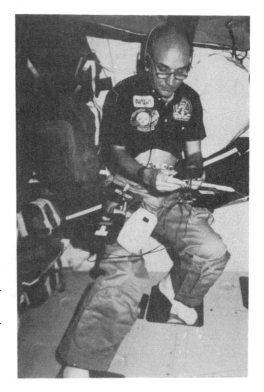

Fig. 25 U.S. Senator E.J. (Jake) Garn conducts a medical experiment on himself in a typical 51-D Garn scene, as the Senator was scheduled as a test subject for extensive medical tests onboard. The particular experiment he is conducting here deals with gastric motility. Principal investigator for this experiment is Astronaut William E. Thornton, a physician (NASA Photo Nos. 85-H-146, 85-HC-121, 51D-10-012).

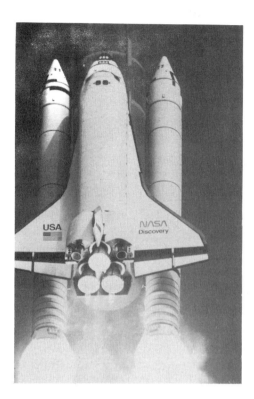

Fig. 26 A low-angle 35mm tracking view of the Space Shuttle Discovery, its external tank and two solid rocket boosters speeding from the KSC launch facility to begin NASA STS 51-G. The camera has captured the diamond shock effect associated with the launch phase or orbiter vehicles. Inside the Discovery are seven crewmembers and a variety of payloads representing international interests. Liftoff for 51-G occurred a 7:33:043 a.m. (EDT), June 17, 1985 (NASA Photo Nos. 85-H-218, 85-HC-189, 51-G(S)-100).

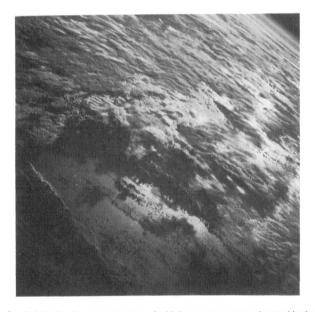

Fig. 27 Sunset over the South Atlantic: As a consequence of a high pressure system located in the South Atlantic, the aerosols generated by fires burning along the coast of West Africa were transported westward. The smoky atmosphere over the South Atlantic produced some of the most beautifully golden sunsets ever witnessed from low Earth orbit (NASA Photo Nos. 85-H-253, 85-HC-224, 51-G-44-092).

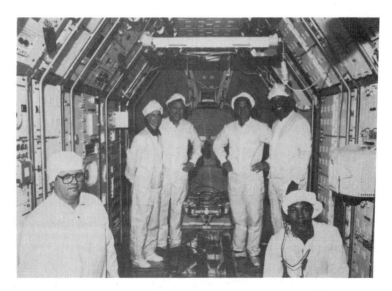

Fig. 28 Standing in the Spacelab D-1, the first payload dedicated to a German mission, four members of the 61-A flight crew prepare to inspect the module containing the Vestibular Sled (VS) prior to launch scheduled for no earlier than October 30, 1985. The VS is an ESA contribution consisting of a seat for a test subject that can be moved backwards and forward with precisely adjusted accelerations along fixed rails on the floor of the Spacelab aisle. The sled permits tests to investigate the functional organization of man's vestibular and orientation system and the vestibular adaptation processes under microgravity. Standing next to the sled, from left to right, are Mission Specialist Bonnie J. Dunbar, Payload Specialists Reinhard Furrer and Ernest Messerschmid and Mission Specialist Guion S. Bluford (NASA Photo Nos. 108-KSC-85PC-442, 85-H-429, 85-HC-389).

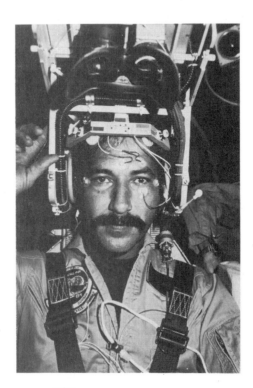

Fig. 29 Dutch Payload Specialist Wubbo J. Ockels on Shuttle flight 61-A prepares to lower the eye-gear portion of the vestibular sled helmet for a test on the busy sled. the scientist has sensors on his face and forehead for systems monitoring (NASA Photo Nos. 85-H-476, 85-HC-430, 61-A-001-023).

163

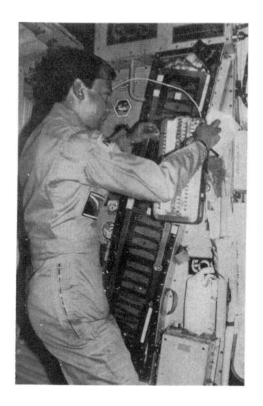

Fig. 30 Charles D. Walker works with the handheld protein crystal growth experiment - one of a series of tests being flown to study the possibility of crystallizing biological materials. Walker rests the experiment against the larger continuous flow electrophoresis systems experiment. Out of frame at right in this 35mm scene is the experiment's control and monitoring unit. Crewmembers for the week-long flight were astronauts Brewster Shaw, Jr., Bryan D. O'Connor, Mary L. Cleave, Sherwood C. Spring, Jerry L. Ross and Payload Specialists Rodolfo Neri of Mexico and Charles D. Walder of McDonnell Douglas. The mission was launched from KSC on November 26 and landed at Edwards Air Force Base on December 3, 1985 (NASA Photo Nos. 85-H-524, 85-HC-473, 61B-02-014).

PUBLICATIONS OF THE
AMERICAN ASTRONAUTICAL SOCIETY

Following are the principal publications of the American Astronautical Society:

JOURNAL OF THE ASTRONAUTICAL SCIENCES (1954-)

Published quarterly and distributed by AAS Business Office, 6212-B Old Keene Mill Court, Springfield, VA 22152. Back issues available from Univelt, Inc., P.O. Box 28130, San Diego, CA 92128.

SPACE TIMES (1986-)

Published bi-monthly and distributed by AAS Business Office, 6212-B Old Keene Mill Court, Springfield, VA 22152., Virginia 22152

AAS NEWSLETTER (1962-1985)

Incorporated in *Space Times*. Back issues available from AAS Business Office, 6212-B Old Keene Mill Court, Springfield, VA 22152.

ASTRONAUTICAL SCIENCES REVIEW (1959-1962)

Incorporated in *Space Times*. Back issues still available from Univelt, Inc., P.O. Box 28130, San Diego, CA 92128.

ADVANCES IN THE ASTRONAUTICAL SCIENCES (1957-)

Proceedings of major AAS technical meetings. Published and distributed for the American Astronautical Society by Univelt, Inc., P.O. Box 28130, San Diego, CA 92128.

SCIENCE AND TECHNOLOGY SERIES (1964-)

Supplement to *Advances in the Astronautical Sciences*. Proceedings and monographs, most of them based on AAS technical meetings. Published and distributed for the American Astronautical Society by Univelt, Inc., P.O. Box 28130, San Diego, CA 92128

AAS HISTORY SERIES (1977-)

Supplement to *Advances in the Astronautical Sciences*. Selected works in the field of aerospace history under the editorship of R. Cargill Hall. Published and distributed for the American Astronautical Society by Univelt, Inc., P.O. Box 28130, San Diego, CA 92128.

AAS MICROFICHE SERIES (1968-)

Supplement to *Advances in the Astronautical Sciences*. Consists principally of technical papers not included in the hard-copy volume. Published and distributed for the American Astronautical Society by Univelt, Inc., P.O. Box 28130, San Diego, CA 92128.

Subscriptions to the *Journal* and the *Space Times* should be ordered from the AAS Business Office. Back issues of the *Journal* and all books and microfiche should be ordered from Univelt, Inc.

SCIENCE AND TECHNOLOGY SERIES (1964-)

ISSN 0278-4017

A **Supplement** to *Advances in the Astronautical Sciences*. **Proceedings and monographs, most of them based on AAS technical meetings.**

Vol. 1   Manned Space Reliability Symposium, Jun. 9, 1964, Anaheim, CA, 1964, 112p., ed. Paul Horowitz, Hard Cover $20 *(ISBN 0-87703-029-4)*

Vol. 2   Towards Deeper Space Penetration (AAS/AAAS Symposium), Dec. 29, 1964, Montreal, Canada, 1964, 182p., ed. Edward R. Van Driest, Hard cover $20 *(ISBN 0-87703-030-8)*

Vol. 3   Orbital Hodograph Analysis, 1965, 150p., ed. Samuel P. Altman, Hard Cover $20 *(ISBN 0-87703-031-6)*

Vol. 4   Scientific Experiments for Manned Orbital Flight, 3rd Goddard Memorial Symposium, Mar. 18-19, 1965, Washington, D.C., 1965, 372p., ed. Peter C. Badgley, Hard Cover $30 *(ISBN 0-87703-032-4)*

Vol. 5   Physiological and Performance Determinants in Manned Space Systems (AAS/HFS Symposium, Apr. 14-15, 1965, Northridge, CA, 1965, 220p., ed. Paul Horowitz, Hard Cover $20 *(ISBN 0-87703-033-2)*

Vol. 6   Space Electronics Symposium (AAS/AES Meeting), May 25-27, 1965, Los Angeles, CA, 1965, 404p., ed. Chung-Ming Wong, Hard Cover $30 *(ISBN 0-87703-034-0)*

Vol. 7   Theodore von Karman Memorial Seminar, May 12, 1965, Los Angeles, CA, 1966, 140p., ed. Shirley Thomas, Hard Cover $30 *(ISBN 0-87703-035-9)*

Vol. 8   Impact of Space Exploration on Society, Aug. 18-20, 1965, San Francisco, CA, 1966, ed. William E. Frye, Hard Cover $30 *(ISBN 0-87703-036-7)*

Vol. 9   Recent Developments in Space Flight Mechanics, (AAS/AAAS Symposium), Dec. 29, 1965, Berkeley, CA, 1966, 280p., ed. Paul B. Richards, Hard Cover $25 *(ISBN 0-87703-037-5)*

Vol. 10   Space in the Fiscal Year 2001, 4th Goddard Memorial Symposium, Mar. 15-16, 1966, Washington, D.C., 1967, 458p., eds. Eugene B. Konecci, Maxwell W. Hunter, II, Robert F. Trapp, Hard Cover $35 *(ISBN 0-87703-038-3)*

Vol. 11   Space Flight Specialist Conference, Jul. 6-8, 1966, Denver, CO, 1967, 618p., ed. Maurice L. Anthony, Hard Cover $45 *(ISBN 0-87703-039-1)*; Microfiche Suppl. (Vol. 2 AAS Microfiche Series) $15 *(ISBN 0-87703-221-1)*

Vol. 12   Management of Aerospace Programs Conference, Nov. 16-18, 1966, Columbia, MO, 1967, 392p., ed. Walter K. Johnson, Hard Cover $30 *(ISBN 0-87703-040-5)*

Vol. 13   Physics of the Moon (AAS/AAAS Symposium), Dec. 29, 1966, Washington, D.C., 1967, 260p., ed. S. Fred Singer, Hard Cover $25 *(ISBN 0-87703-041-3)*

Vol. 14   Interpretation of Lunar Probe Data, Sept. 17, 1966, Huntington Beach, CA, 1967, 270p., ed. Jack Green, Hard Cover $25 *(ISBN 0-87703-042-1)*

Vol. 15   Future Space Program and Impact on Range and Network Development Symposium, Mar. 22-24, 1967, Las Cruces, NM, 1967, 588p., ed. George W. Morgenthaler, Hard Cover $40 *(ISBN 0-87703-043-X)*

Vol. 16   Voyage to the Planets, 5th Goddard Memorial Symposium, Mar. 14-15, 1967, Washington, D.C., 1968, 184p., ed. S. Fred Singer, Hard Cover $20 *(0-87703-044-8)*

Vol. 17   Use of Space Systems for Planetary Geology and Geophysics Symposium, May 25-27, 1967, Boston, MA, 1968, 623p., ed. Robert D. Enzmann, Hard Cover $45 *(ISBN 0-87703-045-6)*; Microfiche Suppl. (Vol. 5 AAS Microfiche Series) $15 *(ISBN 0-87703-135-5)*

Vol. 18 Technology and Social Progress, 6th Goddard Memorial Symposium, Mar. 12-13, 1968, Washington, D.C., 1969, 170p., ed. Philip K. Eckman, Hard Cover $20 *(ISBN 0-87703-046-4)*

Vol. 19 Exobiology - The Search for Extraterrestrial Life (AAS/AAAS Symposium) Dec. 30, 1967, New York, NY, 1969, 184p., eds. Martin M. Freundlich, Bernard W. Wagner, Hard Cover $20 *(ISBN 0-87703-047-2)*

Vol. 20 Bioengineering and Cabin Ecology (AAS/AAAS Symposium) Dec. 30, 1968, Dallas, TX, 1969, 162p., ed. William Cassidy, Hard Cover $20 *(ISBN 0-87703-048-0)*

Vol. 21 Reducing the Cost of Space Transportation, 7th Goddard Memorial Symposium, Mar. 4-5, 1969, Washington, D.C., 1969, 264p., ed. George K. Chacko, Microfiche only $25 *(ISBN 0-87703-049-9)*

Vol. 22 Planning Challenges of the 70's in the Public Domain, 15th Annual AAS Meeting, Jun. 17-20, 1969, Denver, CO, 1970, 504p., eds. William J. Burnsnall, George K. Chacko, George W. Morgenthaler, Hard Cover $40 *(ISBN 0-87703-050-2)*; Microfiche Suppl. (Vol. 13 AAS Microfiche Series) $20 *(ISBN 0-87703-131-2)*; See also Vols. 15-17, AAS Microfiche Series

Vol. 23 Space Technology and Earth Problems Symposium, Oct. 23-25, 1969, Las Cruces, NM, 1970, 418p., ed. C. Quentin Ford, Hard Cover $35 *(ISBN 0-87703-051-0)*; Microfiche Suppl. (Vol. 12 AAS Microfiche Series) $20 *(ISBN 0-87703-134-7)*

Vol. 24 Aerospace Research and Development, Jul. 14, 1966, Holloman AFB, NM, 1970, 500p., ed. Ernst A. Steinhoff, Hard Cover $40 *(ISBN 0-87703-052-9)*

Vol. 25 Geological Problems in Lunar and Planetary Research, Feb. 17-18, 1969, Huntington Beach, CA, 1971, 750p., ed. Jack Green, Hard Cover $45 *(ISBN 0-87703-056-1)*

Vol. 26 Technology Utilization Ideas for the 70s and Beyond, Oct. 30, 1970, Winrock, AR, 1971, 312p., eds. Fred W. Forbes, Paul Dergarabedian, Microfiche only $30 *(ISBN 0-87703-057-X)*

Vol. 27 International Cooperation in Space Operations and Exploration, 9th Goddard Memorial Symposium, Mar. 11, 1971, Washington, D.C. 1971, 194p., ed. Michael Cutler, Hard Cover $20 *(ISBN 0-88703-058-8)*

Vol. 28 Astronomy from a Space Platform (AAS/AAAS Symposium) Dec. 27-28, 1971, Philadelphia, PA, 1972, 416p., eds. George W. Morgenthaler, Howard D. Greyber, Hard Cover $35 *(ISBN 0-87703-061-8)*

Vol. 29 Space Technology Transfer to Community and Industry, 10th Goddard Memorial Symposium, 18th Annual AAS Meeting, Mar. 13-14, 1972, Washington, D.C., 1972, 196p., eds. Ralph H. Tripp, John K. Stotz, Jr., Hard Cover $20 *(ISBN 0-87703-062-6)*; on Microfiche $15

Vol. 30 Space Shuttle Payloads (AAS/AAAS Symposium) Dec. 27-28, 1972, Washington, D.C., 1973, 532p., eds. George W. Morgenthaler, William J. Bursnall, Hard Cover $40 *(ISBN 0-87703-063-4)*

Vol. 31 The Second Fifteen Years in Space, 11th Goddard Memorial Symposium, Mar. 8-9, 1973, Washington, D.C., 1973, 212p., ed. Saul Ferdman, Hard Cover $25 *(ISBN 0-87703-064-2)*

Vol. 32 Health Care Systems Conference, Nov. 21-22, 1972, Dallas, TX, 1974, 265p., ed. Eugene B. Konecci, Hard Cover $25 *(ISBN 0-87703-067-7)*

Vol. 33 Orbital International Laboratory, 3rd and 4th IAF/OIL Symposia, Oct. 5-6, 1970, Constance, Germany, Sept. 24-25, 1971, Brussels, Belgium, 1974, 322p., ed. Ernst A. Steinhoff, Hard Cover $30 *(ISBN 0-87703-068-5)*

Vol. 34 Management and Design of Long-Life Systems, Apr. 24-26, 1973, Denver, CO, 1974, 198p., ed. Harris M. Schurmeier, Hard Cover $20 *(ISBN 0-87703-069-3)*

Vol. 35 Energy Delta, Supply vs. Demand, (AAS/AAAS Symposium) Feb. 25-27, 1974, San Francisco, CA, 1975, 2nd Printing 1976, 604p., eds. George W. Morgenthaler, Aaron N. Silver, Hard Cover $35 *(ISBN 0-87703-070-7)*; Soft Cover $25 *(ISBN 0-87703-082-0)*; on Microfiche $20

Vol. 36 Skylab and Pioneer Report, 12th Goddard Memorial Symposium, Mar. 8, 1974, Washington, D.C., 1975, 160p., eds. Philip H. Bolger, Paul B. Richards, Hard Cover $20 *(ISBN 0-87703-071-5)*

Vol. 37 Space Rescue and Safety 1974, 7th International IAA Symposium, Sept. 30 - Oct. 5, 1974, Amsterdam, Netherlands, 1975, 294p., ed. Philip H. Bolger, Hard Cover $25 *(ISBN 0-87703-073-1)*

Vol. 38 Skylab Science Experiments, (AAS/AAAS Symposium) Feb. 28, 1974, San Francisco, CA, 1976, 274p., eds. George W. Morgenthaler, Gerald E. Simonson, Microfiche only $20 *(ISBN 0-87703-074-X)*

Vol. 39 Environmental Control and Agri-Technology, 1976, 346p., ed. Eugene B. Konecci, Microfiche only $20 *(ISBN 0-87703-075-8)*

Vol. 40 Future Space Activities, 13th Goddard Memorial Symposium, Apr. 11, 1975, Washington, D.C., 1976, 182p., ed. Carl H. Tross, Microfiche only $20 *(ISBN 0-87703-076-6)*

Vol. 41 Space Rescue and Safety 1975, 8th International IAA Symposium, Sept. 21-27, 1975, Lisbon, Portugal, 1976, 230p., ed. Philip H. Bolger, Hard Cover $25 *(ISBN 0-87703-077-4)*

Vol. 42 The End of an Era in Space Exploration, From International Rivalry to International Cooperation, 1976, 216p., by J.C.D. Blaine, Hard Cover $25 *(ISBN 0-87703-084-7)*; without volume number *(ISBN 0-87703-080-4)*

Vol. 43 The Eagle Has Returned, Part I, International Space Hall of Fame Dedication Conference, Oct. 5-9, 1976, Alamogordo, NM, 1976, 370p., ed. Ernst. A. Steinhoff, Hard Cover $30 *(ISBN 0-87703-086-3)*

Vol. 44 Satellite Communications in the Next Decade, 14th Goddard Memorial Symposium, Mar. 12, 1976, Washington, D.C., 1977, 188p., ed. Leonard Jaffe, Hard Cover $20 *(ISBN 0-87703-088-X)*

Vol. 45 The Eagle Has Returned, Part 2, International Space Hall of Fame Dedication Conference, Oct. 5-9, 1976, Alamogordo, NM, 1977, 454p., ed. Ernst A. Steinhoff, Hard Cover $35 *(ISBN 0-87703-092-8)*

Vol. 46 Export of Aerospace Technology, 15th Goddard Memorial Symposium, Mar. 31 - Apr. 1, 1977, Washington, D.C., 1978, 174p., ed. Carl H. Tross, Hard Cover $20 *(ISBN 0-87703-093-6)*

Vol. 47 Handbook of Soviet Lunar and Planetary Exploration, 1979, 276p., by Nicholas L. Johnson, Hard Cover $35 *(ISBN 0-87703-105-3)*; Soft Cover $25 *(ISBN 0-87703-106-1)*

Vol. 48 Handbook of Soviet Manned Space Flight, 2nd Edition, 1988, 474p., by Nicholas L. Johnson, Hard Cover $60 *(ISBN 0-87703-115-0)*; Soft Cover $45 *(ISBN 0-87703-116-9)*

Vol. 49 Space - New Opportunities for International Ventures, 17th Goddard Memorial Symposium, Mar. 28-30, 1979, Washington, D.C., 1980, 300p., ed. William C. Hayes, Jr., Hard over $35 *(ISBN 0-87703-124-X)*; Soft Cover $25 *(ISBN 0-87703-125-8)*; see also Vol. 2 AAS History Series

Vol. 50 Remember the Future - The Apollo Legacy, Jul. 20-21, 1979, San Francisco, CA, 1980, 218p., ed. Stan Kent, Hard Cover $25 *(ISBN 0-87703-126-6)*; Soft Cover $15 *(ISBN 0-87703-127-4)*

Vol. 51 Commercial Operations in Space 1980-2000, 18th Goddard Memorial Symposium, Mar. 27-28, 1980, Washington, D.C., 1981, 214p., eds. John L. McLucas, Charles Sheffield, Hard Cover $30 *(ISBN 0-87703-140-1)*; Soft Cover $20 *(ISBN 0-87703-141-X)*; Microfiche Suppl. (Vol. 34 AAS Microfiche Series) $10 *(ISBN 0-87703-165-7)*; see also Vols. 2 and 3, AAS History Series

Vol. 52 International Space Technical Applications, 19th Goddard Memorial Symposium, Mar. 26-27, 1981, Washington, D.C., 1981, 186p., eds. Andrew Adelman, Peter M. Bainum, Hard Cover $30 *(ISBN 0-87703-152-5)*; Soft Cover $20 *(ISBN 0-87703-153-3)*; see also Vol. 5, AAS History Series

Vol. 53 Space in the 1980's and Beyond, 17th European Space Symposium, Jun. 4-6, 1980, London, England, 1981, 302p., ed. Peter M. Bainum, Hard Cover $40 *(ISBN 0-87703-154-1)*; Soft Cover $30 *(ISBN 0-87703-155-X)*

Vol. 54 Space Safety and Rescue 1979-1981 (with abstracts 1976-1978), Proceedings of symposia of the International Academy of Astronautics held in conjunction with the 30th, 31st, and 32nd International Astronautical Federation Congresses, Munich, Germany, 1979, Tokyo, Japan, 1980, and Rome, Italy, 1981, 1983, 456p., ed. Jeri W. Brown, Hard Cover $45 *(ISBN 0-87703-177-0)*; Soft Cover $35 *(ISBN 0-87703-178-9)*; Microfiche Suppl. (Vols. 39-41 AAS Microfiche Series) $39 *(ISBN 0-87703-222-X)*; *(ISBN 0-87703-223-8)*; *(ISBN 0-87703-224-6)*

Vol. 55 Space Applications at the Crossroads, 21st Goddard Memorial Symposium, Mar. 24-25, 1983, Greenbelt, MD, 1983, 308p., eds. John H. McElroy, E. Larry Heacock, Hard Cover $45 *(ISBN 0-87703-186-X)*; Soft Cover $35 *(ISBN 0-87703-187-8)*

Vol. 56 Space: A Developing Role for Europe, 18th European Space Symposium, Jun. 6-9, 1983, London, England, 1984, 278p., eds. Len J. Carter, Peter M. Bainum, Hard Cover $45 *(ISBN 0-87703-193-2)*; Soft Cover $35 *(ISBN 0-87703-194-0)*; Microfiche Suppl. (Vol. 46 AAS Microfiche Series) $15 *(ISBN 0-87703-195-9)*

Vol. 57 The Case for Mars, Apr. 29 - May 2, 1981, Boulder, CO, 1984, Second Printing 1987, 348p., ed. Penelope J. Boston, Hard Cover $45 *(ISBN 0-87703-197-5)*; Soft Cover $25 *(ISBN 0-87703-198-3)*; on Microfiche $25

Vol. 58 Space Safety and Rescue 1982-1983, Proceedings of the International Academy of Astronautics held in conjunction with the 33rd and 34th International Astronautical Congresses, Paris, France, Sept. 27 - Oct. 2, 1982, and Budapest, Hungary, Oct. 10-15, 1983, 1984, 378p., ed. Gloria W. Heath, Hard Cover $50 *(ISBN 0-87703-202-5)*; Soft Cover $40 *(ISBN 0-87703-203-3)*

Vol. 59 Space and Society - Challenges and Choices, April 14-16, 1982, University of Texas at Austin, 1984, 442p., eds. Paul Anaejionu, Nathan C. Goldman, Philip J. Meeks, Hard Cover $55 *(ISBN 0-87703-204-1)*; Soft Cover $35 *(ISBN 0-87703-205-X)*

Vol. 60 Permanent Presence - Making It Work, 22nd Goddard Memorial Symposium, Mar. 15-16, 1984, Greenbelt, MD, 1985, 190p., ed. Ivan Bekey, Hard Cover $40 *(ISBN 0-87703-207-6)*; Soft Cover $30 *(ISBN 0-87703-208-4)*

Vol. 61 Europe/United States Space Activities - With a Space Propulsion Supplement, 23rd Goddard Memorial Symposium/19th European Space Symposium, Mar. 27-29, 1985, Greenbelt, MD, 31st Annual AAS Meeting, Oct. 22-24, 1984, Palo Alto, CA, 1985, 442p., eds. Peter M. Bainum, Friedrich von Bun, Hard Cover $55 *(ISBN 0-87703-217-3)*; Soft Cover $45 *(ISBN 0-87703-218-1)*

Vol. 62 The Case for Mars II, July 10-14, 1984, Boulder, CO, 1985, 730p., ed. Christopher P. McKay, Hard Cover $60 *(ISBN 0-87703-219-1)*; Soft Cover $40 *(ISBN 0-87703-220-3)*

Vol. 63 Proceedings of 4th International Conference on Applied Numerical Modeling, Dec. 27-29, 1984, Tainan, Taiwan, 1986, 800p., ed. Han-Min Hsia, You-Li Chou, Shu-Yi Wang, Sheng-Jii Hsieh, Hard Cover $70 (ISBN 0-87703-242-4)

Vol. 64 Space Safety and Rescue 1984-1985, Proceedings of the International Academy of Astronautics held in conjunction with the 35th and 36th International Astronautical Congresses, Lausanne, Switzerland, Oct. 7-13, 1984, and Stockholm, Sweden, Oct. 7-12, 1985, 1986, 400p., ed. Gloria W. Heath, Hard Cover $55 *(ISBN 0-87703-248-3)*; Soft Cover $45 *(ISBN 0-87703-249-1)*

Vol. 65 The Human Quest in Space, 24th Goddard Memorial Symposium, Mar. 20-21, 1986, Greenbelt, MD, 1987, 312p., ed. Gerald L. Burdett, Gerald A. Soffen, Hard Cover $55 *(ISBN 0-87703-262-9)*; Soft Cover $45 *(ISBN 0-87703-263-7)*

Vol. 66 Soviet Space Programs 1980-1985, 1987, 298p., by Nicholas L. Johnson, Hard Cover $55 *(ISBN 0-87703-266-1)*; Soft Cover $45 *(ISBN 0-87703-267-X)*

Vol. 67 Low-Gravity Sciences, Seminar Series 1986, University of Colorado at Boulder, 290p., ed. Jean N. Koster, Hard Cover $55 *(ISBN 0-87703-270-X)*; Soft Cover $45 *(ISBN 0-87703-271-8)*

Vol. 68 Proceedings of the Fourth Annual L5 Space Development Conference, Apr. 25-28, 1985, Washington, D.C., 1987, 268p., ed. Frank Hecker, Hard Cover $50 *(ISBN 0-87703-272-6)*; Soft Cover $35 *(ISBN 0-87703-273-4)*

Vol. 69 Visions of Tomorrow: A Focus on National Space Transportation Issues, 25th Goddard Memorial Symposium, Mar. 18-20, 1987, Greenbelt, MD, 1987, 338p., ed. Gerald A. Soffen, Hard Cover $55 *(ISBN 0-87703-274-2)*; Soft Cover $45 *(ISBN 0-87703-275-0)*

Vol. 70 Space Safety and Rescue 1986-1987, Proceedings of the International Academy of Astronautics held in conjunction with the 37th and 38th International Astronautical Congresses, Innsbruck, Austria, Oct. 4-11, 1986, and Brighton, England, Oct. 11-16, 1987, 1988, 360p., ed. Gloria W. Heath, Hard Cover $55 *(ISBN 0-87703-291-2)*; Soft Cover $45 *(ISBN 0-87703-292-0)*

Vol. 71 The NASA Mars Conference, Jul. 21-23, 1986, Washington, D.C., 1988, 570p., ed. Duke B. Reiber, Hard Cover $50 *(ISBN 0-87703-293-9)*; Soft Cover $30 *(ISBN 0-87703-294-7)*

Vol. 72 Working in Orbit and Beyond: The Challenges for Space Medicine, Jun. 20-21, 1987, Washington, D.C., 1989, 188p., ed. David Lorr, Victoria Garshnek, Hard Cover $45 *(ISBN 0-87703-295-5)*; Soft Cover $35 *(ISBN 0-87703-296-3)*

Order from Univelt, Inc., P.O. Box 28130, San Diego, California 92128

ADVANCES IN THE ASTRONAUTICAL SCIENCES SERIES (1957-)

ISSN 0065-3438, LIBRARY OF CONGRESS CARD NO. 57-43769

Proceedings of Major AAS Technical Meetings

Vol. 1 Third Annual AAS Meeting, Dec. 6-7, 1956, New York, NY, 1957, 184p., ed. Norman V. Petersen, Microfiche only, $20 *(ISBN 0-87703-002-2)*

Vol. 2 Fourth Annual AAS Meeting, Jan. 29-31, 1958, New York, NY, 1958, 440p., eds. Norman V. Petersen, Horace Jacobs, Microfiche only, $20 *(ISBN 0-87703-003-0)*

Vol. 3 First Western National AAS Meeting, Aug. 18-19, 1958 530p., eds. Norman V. Petersen, Horace Jacobs, Microfiche only, $20 *(ISBN 0-87703-004-9)*

Vol. 4 Fifth Annual AAS Meeting, Dec. 27-31, 1958, Washington, D.C., 1959, 462p., ed. Horace Jacobs, Microfiche only, $20 *(ISBN 0-87703-005-7)*

Vol. 5 Second Western National AAS Meeting, Aug. 4-5, 1959, Los Angeles, CA, 1960, 364p., ed. Horace Jacobs, Microfiche only, $20 *(ISBN 0-87703-006-3)*

Vol. 6 Sixth Annual AAS Meeting, Jan. 18-21, 1960, New York, NY, 1961, 968p., eds. Horace Jacobs and Eric Burgess, Hard Cover $45 *(ISBN 0-87703-007-3)*

Vol. 7 Third Western National AAS Meeting, Aug. 4-5, 1960, Seattle, WA, 1961, 464p., eds. Horace Jacobs and Eric Burgess, Microfiche only, $20 *(ISBN 0-87703-008-1)*

Vol. 8 Seventh Annual AAS Meeting, Jan. 16-18, 1961, Dallas, TX, 1963, 602p., ed. Horace Jacobs, Microfiche only, $20 *(ISBN 0-87703-009-X)*

Vol. 9 Fourth Western Regional AAS Meeting, Aug. 1-3, 1961, San Francisco, CA, 1963, 910p., ed. Eric Burgess, Hard Cover $45 *(ISBN 0-87703-010-3)*

Vol. 10 Manned Lunar Flight (AAS/AAAS Symposium) Dec. 19, 1961, Denver, CO, 1963, 310p., eds. George W. Morgenthaler and Horace Jacobs, Hard Cover $35 *(ISBN 0-87703-011-1)*

Vol. 11 Eighth Annual AAS Meeting, Jan. 16-18, 1962, Washington, D.C., 1963, 808p., ed. Horace Jacobs, Hard Cover $45 *(ISBN 0-87703-012-X)*

Vol. 12 Scientific Satellites - Mission and Design (AAS/AAAS Symposium), Dec. 27, 1962, Philadelphia, PA, 1963, 262p., ed. Irving E. Jeter, Hard Cover $25 *(ISBN 0-87703-013-8)*

Vol. 13 Interplanetary Missions, 9th Annual AAS Meeting, Jan. 15-17, 1963, Los Angeles, CA, 1963, 690p., ed. Eric Burgess, Hard Cover $45 *(ISBN 0-87703-014-6)*

Vol. 14 Second AAS Symposium on Physical and Biological Phenomena under Zero G Conditions, Jan. 18, 1963, Los Angeles, CA, 1963, 382p., eds. Elliot T. Benedikt and Robert W. Halliburton, Hard Cover $30 *(ISBN 0-87703-015-4)*

Vol. 15 Exploration of Mars Symposium, Jun. 6-7, 1963, Denver, CO, 1963, 634p., ed. George W. Morgenthaler, Hard Cover $45 *(ISBN 0-87703-016-2)*

Vol. 16 Space Rendezvous, Rescue, and Recovery Symposium, Sept. 10-12, 1963, Edwards, CA 1963, 1408p., ed. Norman V. Petersen, Hard Cover, **Part 1**, 1028p., $45 *(ISBN 0-87703-017-0)*; **Part 2**, 380p., $30 *(ISBN 0-87703-018-9)*

Vol. 17 Bioastronautics - Fundamental and Practical Problems (AAS/AAAS Symposium), Dec. 30, 1963, Cleveland, OH, 1964, 128p., ed. William C. Kaufman, Microfiche only, $10 *(ISBN 0-87703-019-7)*

Vol. 18 Lunar Flight Programs, 10th Annual AAS Meeting, May 4-7, 1964, New York, NY, 1964, 630p., ed. Ross Fleisig, Hard Cover $45 *(ISBN 0-87703-020-0)*

Vol. 19 Unmanned Exploration of the Solar System Symposium, Feb. 8-10, 1965, Denver, CO, 1965, 1000p., eds. George W. Morgenthaler, Robert G. Morra, Hard Cover $45 *(ISBN 0-87703-021-9)*

Vol. 20 Post Apollo Exploration, 11th Annual AAS Meeting, May 3-6, 1965, Chicago, IL, 1966, 1220p., ed. Francis Narin, Microfiche only, **Part I**, 572p., $30 *(ISBN 0-87703-022-7)*; **Part 2**, 648p., $35 *(ISBN 0-87703-023-5)*

Vol. 21 Practical Space Applications Symposium, Feb. 21-23, 1966, San Diego, CA, 1967, 508p., ed. Lawrence L. Kavanau, Hard Cover $40 *(ISBN 0-87703-024-3)*

Vol. 22 The Search for Extraterrestrial Life, 12th Annual AAS Meeting, May 23-25, 1966, Anaheim, CA, 1967, 388p., ed. James S. Hanrahan, Microfiche only $30 *(ISBN 0-87703-025-1)*; Microfiche Suppl. (Vol. 1 AAS Microfiche Series) $12 *(ISBN 0-87703-132-0)*

Vol. 23 Commercial Utilization of Space, 13th Annual AAS Meeting, May 1-3, 1967, Dallas, TX, 1968, 512p., eds. J. Ray Gilmer, Alfred M. Mayo, Ross C. Peavey, Hard Cover *(ISBN 0-87703-026-X)*; plus Microfiche Suppl. (Vol. 3 AAS Microfiche Series) $60 *(ISBN 0-87703-216-5)*

Vol. 24 Exploitation of Space for Experimental Research, 14th Annual AAS Meeting, May 13-15, 1968, Dedham, MA, 1968, 363p., ed. Harry Zuckerberg, Hard Cover $30 *(ISBN 0-87703-027-8)*

Vol. 25 Advanced Space Experiments, Sept. 16-18, 1968, Ann Arbor, MI, 1969, 530p., eds. O. Lyle Tiffany and Eugene M. Zaitzeff, Hard Cover $40 *(ISBN 0-87703-028-6)*

Vol. 26 Planning Challenges of the 70's in Space, 15th Annual AAS Meeting, Jun. 17-20, 1969, Denver, CO, 1970, 470p., eds. George W. Morgenthaler and Robert G. Morra, Hard Cover $35 *(ISBN 0-87703-053-7)*; Microfiche Suppl. (Vol. 14 AAS Microfiche Series) $20 *(ISBN 0-87703-130-4)*

Vol. 27/28 Space Stations (**v27**) and Space Shuttles and Interplanetary Missions (**v28**), 16th Annual AAS Meeting, Jun. 8-10, 1970, Anaheim, CA, 1970, **Vol. 27**, eds. Lewis Larmore and Robert L. Gervais, 6060p., Hard Cover $45 *(ISBN 0-87703-054-5)*; **Vol. 28**, eds. Lewis Larmore and Robert L. Gervais, 488p., Hard Cover $35 *(ISBN 0-87703-055-3)*

Vol. 29 The Outer Solar System, 17th Annual AAS Meeting, Jun. 28-30, 1971, Seattle, WA, 1971, 1358p., $85; ed. Juris Vagners, Hard Cover, **Part 1**, 618p., $40 *(ISBN 0-87703-059-6)*; **Part 2**, 740p., $45 *(ISBN 0-87703-060-X)*

Vol. 30 International Congress of Space Benefits, 19th Annual AAS Meeting, Jun. 19-21, 1973, Dallas, TX, 1974, 528p., ed. Francis S. Johnson, Hard Cover $40 *(ISBN 0-87703-065-0)*

Vol. 31 The Skylab Results, 20th Annual AAS Meeting, Aug. 20-22, 1974, Los Angeles, CA, 1975, 1174p., eds. William C. Schneider and Thomas E. Hanes, Microfiche only (ISBN 0-87703-072-3); Plus Microfiche Suppl. (Vol. 22 AAS Microfiche Series) $60 *(ISBN 0-87703-043-6)*

Vol. 32 Space Shuttle Missions of the 80's, 21st Annual AAS Meeting, Aug. 26-28, 1975, Denver, CO, 1977, 1364p., eds. William J. Bursnall, George W. Morgenthaler, Gerald E. Simonson, Hard Cover, **Part 1**, 598p., $40 *(ISBN 0-87703-078-2)*; Hard Cover, **Part 2**, 766p., $55 *(ISBN 0-87703-087-1)*; Microfiche Suppl. (Vol. 25 AAS Microfiche Series $65 *(ISBN 0-87703-133-9)*

Vol. 33 AAS/AIAA Astrodynamics Conference, July 28-30, 1975, Nassau, Bahamas, 1976, 390p., eds. William F. Powers, Herbert E. Rauch, Byron D. Tapley, Carmelo E. Velez, Hard Cover $35 *(ISBN 0-87703-079-0)*; Microfiche Suppl. (Vol. 26 AAS Microfiche Series) $40 *(ISBN 0-87703-142-8)*

Vol. 34 Apollo Soyuz Mission Report, 1977, 336p., ed. Chester M. Lee, Hard Cover $35 *(ISBN 0-87703-089-8)*

Vol. 35 The Bicentennial Space Symposium - New Themes for Space: Mankind's Future Needs and Aspirations, 22nd AAS Meeting, Oct. 6-8, 1976, Washington, D.C., 1977, 242p., ed. William C. Schneider, Hard Cover $25 *(ISBN 0-87703-090-1)*

Vol. 36 The Industrialization of Space, 23rd Annual AAS Meeting, Oct. 18-20, 1977, San Francisco, CA, 1978, 1160p., eds. Richard A. Van Patten, Paul Siegler, Edward V.B. Stearns, Hard Cover, **Part 1**, 610p., $55 *(ISBN 0-87703-094-4)*; Hard Cover, **Part 2**, 550p., $45 *(ISBN 0-87703-095-2)*; Microfiche Suppl. (Vol. 28 AAS Microfiche Series) $15 *(ISBN 0-87703-121-5)*

Vol. 37 Space Shuttle and Spacelab Utilization, What are the Near-Term and Long-Term Benefits for Mankind?, 16th Goddard Memorial Symposium, 24th Annual AAS Meeting, March 8-10, 1978, Washington, D.C., 1978, 865p., eds. George W. Morgenthaler and Manfred Hollstein, Hard Cover, **Part 1**, 400p., $40 *(ISBN 0-87703-096-0)*; Hard Cover, **Part 2**, 465p., $45 *(ISBN 0-87703-097-9)*

Vol. 38 The Future U.S. Space Program, 25th Anniversary Conference, Oct. 20 - Nov. 2, 1978, Houston, TX, 1979, 880p., eds. Richard S. Johnston, Albert Naumann, Jr., Clay W. G. Fulcher, Hard Cover, **Part 1**, 444p., $45 *(ISBN 0-87703-098-7)*; Hard Cover, **Part 2**, 436p., $40 *(ISBN 0-87703-099-5)*; Microfiche Suppl. (Vol. 30 AAS Microfiche Series) $15 *(ISBN 0-87703-129-0)*

Vol. 39 Guidance and Control 1979, Feb. 24-28, 1979, Keystone, CO, 1979, 492p., ed. Robert D. Culp, Hard Cover $45 *(ISBN 0-87703-100-2)*; Microfiche Suppl. (Vol. 31 AAS Microfiche Series) $10 *(ISBN 0-87703-128-2)*

Vol. 40 AAS/AIAA Astrodynamics Conference, Jun. 25-27, 1979, Provincetown, MA, 1980, 996p., eds. Paul A. Penzo, Bernard Kaufman, Louis Friedman, Richard Battin, Hard Cover, **Part 1**, 494p., $45 *(ISBN 0-87703-107-X)*; Soft Cover $35 *(ISBN 0-87703-108-8)*; Hard Cover, **Part 2**, 502p., $45 *(ISBN 0-87703-109-6)*; Soft Cover $35 *(ISBN 0-87703-110-X)*; Microfiche Suppl. (Vol. 32 AAS Microfiche Series) $20 *(ISBN 0-87703-139-8)*

Vol. 41 Space Shuttle: Dawn of an Era, 26th Annual AAS Meeting, Oct. 29-Nov. 1, 1979, Los Angeles, CA, 1980, 980p., eds. William F. Rector, III and Paul A. Penzo, Hard Cover, **Part 1**, 452p., $45 *(ISBN 0-87703-111-8)*; Soft Cover $35 *(ISBN 0-87703-112-6)*; Hard Cover, **Part 2**, 528p., $55 *(ISBN 0-87703-113-4)*; Soft Cover $40 *(ISBN 0-87703-114-2)*; Microfiche Suppl. (Vol. 33 AAS Microfiche Series) $10 *(ISBN 0-87703-136-3)*

Vol. 42 Guidance and Control 1980, Feb. 17-21, 1980, Keystone, CO, 1980, 738p., ed. Louis A. Morine, Hard Cover $60 *(ISBN 0-87703-137-1)*; Soft Cover $45 *(ISBN 0-87703-138-X)*

Vol. 43 Shuttle/Spacelab - The New Transportation System and its Utilization, (3rd DGLR/AAS Symposium), Apr. 28-30, 1980, Hannover, Germany, 1981, 342p., eds. Dietrich E. Koelle and George V. Butler, Hard Cover $45 *(ISBN 0-87703-144-4)*; Soft Cover $35 *(ISBN 0-87703-146-0)*

Vol. 44 Space--Enhancing Technological Leadership, 27th Annual AAS Meeting, Oct. 20-23, 1980, Boston, MA, 1981, 580p., ed. Lawrence P. Greene, Hard Cover $65 *(ISBN 0-87703-147-9)*; Soft Cover $50 *(ISBN 0-87703-148-7)*; Microfiche Suppl. (Vol. 35 AAS Microfiche Series) $10 *(ISBN 0-87703-164-9)*

Vol. 45 Guidance and Control 1981, Jan. 31- Feb. 4, 1981, Keystone, CO, 1981, 506p., ed. Edward J. Bauman, Hard Cover $60 *(ISBN 0-87703-150-9)*; Soft Cover $50 *(ISBN 0-87703-151-7)*; Microfiche Suppl. (Vol. 36 AAS Microfiche Series) $15 *(ISBN 0-87703-156-8)*

Vol. 46 AAS/AIAA Astrodynamics Conference, Aug. 3-5, 1981, North Lake Tahoe, NV, 1982, 1124p., eds. Alan L. Friedlander, Paul J. Cefola, Bernard Kaufman, Walt Williamson, G.T. Tseng, Hard Cover, **Part 1**, 552p., $55 *(ISBN 0-87703-159-2)*; Soft Cover $45 *(ISBN 0-87703-160-6)*; Hard Cover, **Part 2**, 572p., $55 *(ISBN 0-87703-161-4)*; Soft Cover $45 *(ISBN 0-87703-162-2)*; Microfiche Suppl. (Vol. 37 AAS Microfiche Series) $40 *(ISBN 0-87703-163-0)*

Vol. 47 Leadership in Space - For Benefits on Earth, 28th Annual AAS Meeting, Oct. 26-29, 1981, San Diego, CA, 1982, 310p., ed. William F. Rector, III, Hard Cover $45 *(ISBN 0-87703-168-1)*; Soft Cover $35 *(ISBN 0-87703-169-X)*

Vol. 48 Guidance And Control 1982, Jan. 30 - Feb. 3, 1982, Keystone, CO, 1982, 558p., eds. Robert D. Culp, Edward J. Bauman, W. E. Dorroh, Jr., Hard Cover $65 *(ISBN 0-87703-170-3)*; Soft Cover $50 *(ISBN 0-87703-171-1)*; Microfiche Suppl. (Vol. 38 AAS Michrofiche Series) $10 *(ISBN 0-87703-180-0)*

Vol. 49 Spacelab, Space Platforms, and the Future, Fourth AAS/DGLR Symposium and 20th Goddard Memorial Symposium, Mar. 17-19, 1982, Greenbelt, MD, 1982, 502p., eds. Peter M. Bainum, Dietrich E. Koelle, Hard Cover $55 *(ISBN 0-87703-174-6)*; Soft Cover $45 *(ISBN 0-87703-175-4)*; Microfiche Suppl. (Vol. 42 AAS Microfiche Series) $15 *(ISBN 0-87703-181-9)*

Vol. 50 Proceedings on an International Symposium on Engineering Sciences and Mechanics, Dec. 29-31, Tainan, Taiwan, 1983, **two parts**, 1570p., eds. Han-Min Hsia, Richard W. Longman, You-Li Chou, Hard Cover $120 *(ISBN 0-87703-176-2)*; Microfiche Suppl. (Vol. 43 AAS Microfiche Series) $10 *(ISBN 0-87703-215-7)*

Vol. 51 Guidance and Control 1983, Feb. 5-9, 1983, Keystone, CO, 1983, 494p., eds. Edward J. Bauman, Zubin W. Emsley, Hard Cover $60 *(ISBN 0-87703-182-7)*; Soft Cover $50 *(ISBN 0-87703-183-5)*; Microfiche Suppl. (Vol. 44 AAS Microfiche Series) $10 *(ISBN 0-87703-214-9)*

Vol. 52 Developing the Space Frontier, 29th Annual AAS Meeting, Oct. 25-27, 1982, Houston, TX, 1983, 436p., eds. Albert Naumann, Grover Alexander, Hard Cover $55 *(ISBN 0-87703-189-4)*

Vol. 53 Space Manufacturing 1983, May 9-12, 1983, Princeton, NJ, 1983, 496p., eds. James D. Burke, April S. Whitt, Hard Cover $60 *(ISBN 0-87703-188-6)*; Soft Cover $50 *(0-87703-189-4)*

Vol. 54 AAS/AIAA Astrodynamics Conference, Aug. 22-25, 1983, Lake Placid, NY, 1984, **two parts**, 1370p., eds. G.T. Tseng, Paul J. Cefola, Peter M. Bainum, David A. Levinson, Hard Cover $120 *(ISBN 0-87703-190-8)*; Soft Cover $90 *(ISBN 0-87703-191-6)*; Microfiche Suppl. (Vol. 45 AAS Microfiche Series) $40 *(ISBN 0-87703-192-4)*

Vol. 55 Guidance and Control 1984, Feb. 4-8, 1984, Keystone, CO, 1984, 500p., eds. Robert D. Culp, Parker S. Stafford, Hard Cover $60 *(ISBN 0-87703-199-1)*; Soft Cover $50 *(ISBN 0-87703-200-9)*; Microfiche Suppl. (Vol. 48 AAS Microfiche Series $15 *(ISBN 0-87703-201-7)*

Vol. 56 From Spacelab to Space Station, Fifth DGLR/AAS Symposium, Oct. 3-5, 1984, Hamburg, Germany, 1985, 270p., eds. H. Stoewer, Peter M. Bainum, Microfiche Only $30 *(ISBN 0-87703-209-2)*

Vol. 57 Guidance and Control 1985, Feb. 2-6, 1985, Keystone, CO, 1985, 618p., eds. Robert D. Culp, Edward J. Bauman, Charles A. Cullian, Hard Cover $65 *(ISBN 0-87703-211-4)*; Soft Cover $50 *(ISBN 0-87703-212-2)*; Microfiche Suppl. (Vol. 50 AAS Microfiche Series) $15 *(ISBN 0-87703-213-0)*

Vol. 58 AAS/AIAA Astrodynamics Conference, Aug. 12-15, 1985, Vail, CO, 1986, **two parts**, 1556p., eds. Bernard Kaufman, Joseph J.F. Liu, Robert A. Calico, Felix R. Hoots, Hard Cover $140 *(ISBN 0-87703-245-9)*; Soft Cover $110 *(ISBN 0-87703-246-7)*; Microfiche Suppl. (Vol. 51 AAS Microfiche Series); $60 *(ISBN 0-87703-247-5)*

Vol. 59 Space Station Beyond IOC, 32nd Annual AAS Meeting, Nov 6-7, 1985, Los Angeles, CA, 1986, 188p., ed. M. Jack Friedenthal, Hard Cover $40 *(ISBN 0-87703-252-1)*; Soft Cover $30 *(ISBN 0-87703-253-X)*

Vol. 60 Space Exploitation and Utilization, First AAS/JRS Symposium, Dec. 15-19, 1985, Honolulu, HI, 1986, 740p., eds. Gayle L. May, Peter M. Bainum, Kenji Ikeda, Tamiya Nomura, Tatsuo Yamanaka, Ryojiro Akiba, Hard Cover $70 *(ISBN 0-87703-254-8)*; Soft Cover $55 *(ISBN 0-87703-255-6)*; Microfiche Suppl. (Vol. 52 AAS Microfiche Series) $10 *(ISBN 0-87703-256-4)*

Vol. 61 Guidance and Control 1986, Feb. 1-5, 1986, Keystone, CO, 1986, 460p., eds. Robert D. Culp, John C. Durrett, Hard Cover $60 *(ISBN 0-87703-257-2)*; Soft Cover $50 *(ISBN 0-87703-258-0)*; Microfiche Suppl. (Vol. 53 AAS Microfiche Series) $10 *(ISBN 0-87703-259-9)*

Vol. 62 Tethers in Space, Proceedings of First International Conference on Tethers in Space (NASA & PSN Sponsors; AIAA, AAS, & AIDAA Co-Sponsors), Sept. 17-19, 1986, Arlington, VA, 1987, 784p., eds. Peter M. Bainum, Ivan Bekey, Luciano Guerriero, Paul A. Penzo, Hard Cover $80 *(ISBN 0-87703-264-5)*; Soft Cover $70 *(ISBN 0-87703-265-3)*

Vol. 63 Guidance and Control 1987, Jan. 31 - Feb. 4, 1987, Keystone, CO, 1987, 638p., eds. Robert D. Culp, Terry J. Kelly, Hard Cover $75 *(ISBN 0-87703-268-8)*; Soft Cover $60 *(ISBN 0-87703-269-6)*

Vol. 64 Aerospace Century XXI, 33rd AAS Annual Meeting, Oct. 26-29, 1986, Boulder, CO, 1987, **all three parts**, Hard Cover $225 *(ISBN 0-87703-276-9)*; Soft Cover $180 *(ISBN 0-87703-277-7)*; **Part I**, Space Missions and Policy, 686p., eds. George W. Morgenthaler, Gayle L. May, Hard Cover $75 *(ISBN 0-87703-279-3)*; Soft Cover $60 *(ISBN 0-87703-282-3)*; **Part II**, Space Flight Technologies, 608p., eds. George W. Morgenthaler, W. Kent Tobiska, Hard Cover $75 *(ISBN 0-87703-280-7)*; Soft Cover $60 *(ISBN 0-87703-283-1)*; **Part III**, Space Sciences, Applications, and Commercial Developments, 724p., eds. George W. Morgenthaler, Jean N. Koster, Hard Cover $75 *(ISBN 0-87703-281-5)*; Soft Cover $60 *(ISBN 0-87703-284-X)*; Microfiche Suppl. (Vol. 54 AAS Microfiche Series) $25 *(ISBN 0-87703-278-5)*

Vol. 65 AAS/AIAA Astrodynamics Conference, Aug. 10-13, 1987, Kalispell, MT, 1988, **two parts**, 1774p., eds. John K. Soldner, Arun K. Misra, Robert E. Lindberg, Walton Williamson, Hard Cover $180 *(ISBN 0-87703-285-8)*; Soft Cover $150 *(ISBN 0-87703-286-6)*; Microfiche Suppl. (Vol. 55 AAS Microfiche Series); $70 *(ISBN 0-87703-287-4)*

Vol. 66 Guidance and Control 1988, Jan. 30 - Feb. 3, 1988, Keystone, CO, 1988, 576p., eds. Robert D. Culp, Paul L. Shattuck, Hard Cover $75 *(ISBN 0-87703-288-2)*; Soft Cover $60 *(ISBN 0-87703-289-0)*; Microfiche Suppl. (Vol. 56 AAS Microfiche Series) $10 *(ISBN 0-87703-290-4)*

Vol. 67 Space - A New Community of Opportunity, 34th AAS Annual Meeting, Nov. 3-5, 1987, Houston, TX, 1989, approx. 500p., ed. William G. Straight, Henry N. Bowes, Hard Cover $70 *(ISBN 0-87703-297-1)*; Soft Cover $55 *(ISBN 0-87703-298-X)*

Order from Univelt, Inc., P.O. Box 28130, San Diego, California 92128

INDEX

Available in two volumes is an INDEX TO ALL AMERICAN
ASTRONAUTICAL SOCIETY PAPERS AND ARTICLES 1954-1985

This index is a numerical/chronological index (which also serves
as a citation index) and an author index. (A subject index volume
will be forthcoming in 1987.)

It covers all articles that appear in the following:

Advances in the Astronautical Sciences (1957-August 1986)

Science and Technology Series (1964-September 1986)

AAS History Series (1977-1986)

AAS Microfiche Series (1968-August 1986)

Journal of the Astronautical Sciences (1954-March 1986)

Astronautical Sciences Review (1959-1962)

If you are in aerospace you will want this excellent reference
tool which covers the first 30 years of the Space Age.

Numerical/Chronological/Author Index in two volumes, Library
Binding (both volumes) $95; Soft Cover (both Volumes) $80;
Volume I (1954-1978) Library Binding $40; Soft Cover $30;
Volume II (1979-1985/86) Library Binding $60; Soft Cover $45.
Order from Univelt, Inc., P.O. Box 28130, San Diego,
California 92128.

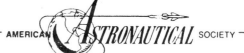

AMERICAN *ASTRONAUTICAL* SOCIETY

NUMERICAL INDEX

AUTHOR INDEX[*]

---

[*] For each author the AAS paper number is given. The page numbers refer to Volume 72, <u>Science and Technology Series</u>.